ARTIFICIAL INSEMINATION IN ANIMALS

ARTIFICIAL INSEMINATION
in Animals

William Morris
Emily Root

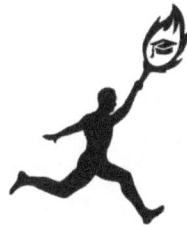

Kruger Brentt
Publishers

2023

Kruger Brentt Publishers UK. LTD.
Company Number 9728962

Regd. Office: 68 St Margarets Road, Edgware, Middlesex HA8 9UU

© 2023 AUTHORS
ISBN: 9781787150393

For information on all our publications visit our website at http://krugerbrentt.com/

PREFACE

Artificial insemination (AI) is the manual placement of semen in the reproductive tract of the female by a method other than natural mating. It is one of a group of technologies commonly known as "assisted reproduction technologies" (ART), whereby offspring are generated by facilitating the meeting of gametes (spermatozoa and oocytes). ART may also involve the transfer of the products of conception to a female, for instance if fertilization has taken place in vitro or in another female. Other techniques encompassed by ART include the following: in vitro fertilization (IVF) where fertilization takes place outside the body; intracytoplasmic sperm injection (ICSI) where a single spermatozoon is caught and injected into an oocyte; embryo transfer (ET) where embryos that have been derived either in vivo or in vitro are transferred to a recipient female to establish a pregnancy; gamete intrafallopian transfer (GIFT) where spermatozoa are injected into the oviduct to be close to the site of fertilization in vivo; and cryopreservation, where spermatozoa or embryos, or occasionally oocytes, are cryopreserved in liquid nitrogen for use at a later stage. AI has been used in the majority of domestic species, including bees, and also in human beings. It is the most commonly used ART in livestock, revolutionising the animal breeding industry during the 20th century. In contrast to medical use, where intra-uterine insemination (IUI) is used only occasionally in human fertility treatment, AI is by far the most common method of breeding intensively kept domestic livestock, such as dairy cattle, pigs and turkeys (almost 100% in intensive production). AI is increasing in horses, beef cattle and sheep, and has been reported in other domestic species such as dogs, goats, deer and buffalo. It has also been used occasionally in conservation breeding of rare or endangered species, for example, primates, elephants and wild felids.

The present book contains Twenty three chapters covering all related disciplines. These chapters include introduction to artificial insemination, anatomy of the reproductive tracts, fixed time ai protocols: a tool for effective reproductive management of dairy animals, artificial insemination: current and future trends, semen quality and fertility after artificial insemination, artificial insemination and embryo transfer in goats, canine artificial insemination, dairy genetic improvement and artificial insemination, advances in cryopreservation of bull sperm, artificial insemination in poultry, laparoscopic artificial insemination technique in small ruminants, problems of artificial insemination in dromedarius camel - failure of ovulation and cryoprotectants & cryopreservation of equine semen. Related terminology is given at the end for ready reference. This book deals with some of the emerging topics on advanced concepts in artificial insemination, which would an invaluable asset for the scientists, students and teachers working in the field of animal science, veterinary science animal and human genetics. This book is also a valuable reference source for anyone interested in knowing more about advanced concepts in artificial insemination.

We are grateful to all those persons as well as various books, manuals, periodicals, magazines, journals etc. that helped in the preparation of this book. In spite of the best efforts, it is possible that some errors may have occurred into the compilation and editing of the book. Further queries, constructive suggestions and criticisms for the improvement of the book are always welcome and shall be thankfully acknowledged

William Morris
Emily Root

CONTENTS

1

INTRODUCTION TO ARTIFICIAL INSEMINATION

1.1 INTRODUCTION: AN OVERVIEW

The rationale behind artificial insemination is increasing the gamete density at the site of fertilization. Since many centuries different pioneers contributed to the history of artificial insemination, not only in humans but even more pronounced in farm animals. The primary reason for using this technique in farm animals was to speed up the rate of genetic improvement by increasing the productivity of food producing animals. This was accomplished by improving the selection differential wherein one highly selected male is mated with thousands of females. The AID industry was born.

Good productions as well as good reproduction are two essential elements for making the dairy farming/business a profitable one. A number of new reproductive technologies have been implemented for enhancing reproductive performances of dairy animals. Artificial insemination is one of the most important reproductive technologies implemented by the dairy industry. Artificial Insemination (AI) is very useful in a country like India where the availability of quality males (sires) is inadequate and has become the major hurdle in the way of dairy animals' development.

- For humans the situation is different: artificial insemination was originally developed to help couples to conceive in case of severe male factor sub-fertility of a physical or psychological nature. Nowadays artificial insemination with homologous semen is most commonly used for unexplained and mild male factor sub-fertility. In the previous century donor insemination was mainly used for male infertility due to azoospermia or very low sperm count and for inherited genetic diseases linked to the Y-chromosome. Nowadays donor insemination is more commonly used in women with no male partner (lesbians or single women).

- Artificial insemination (AI) is a method of breeding cattle using frozen straws of semen. In order for the process to be successful it must be done at the proper time of a cow's heat cycle. In the past this required observing cows for heat in order to breed at the appropriate time. However, the most common method of AI today uses a synchronization protocol to bring the majority of the herd into heat at the same time so they can be bred using timed AI. Improvements in synchronization techniques has made artificial insemination a much more feasible option for today's cattle producers.

1.2 MILESTONES IN THE HISTORY OF ARTIFICIAL INSEMINATION

Unofficial history claims that the first attempts to artificially inseminate a woman, were done by Henry IV (1425-1474), King of Castile, nicknamed the Impotent. In 1455, he married Princess Juana, sister of Afonso V of Portugal. After six years of marriage she gave birth to a daughter, Joanna. Many contemporary historians and chroniclers assumed Henry was impotent. The possibility of artificial insemination was launched. Later on it was claimed that the princess was not the daughter of the king.

Spermatozoa were first seen and described by **Antoni van Leeuwenhoek** and his assistant **Johannes Ham** in 1678 in the Netherlands. In a letter to William Bounker of the Royal Society of London (Phil.Trans. Vol.XII, nbr. 142, 1678) he showed a picture of sperm cells of the human and the dog. van Leeuwenhoek described the spermatozoa as "zaaddiertjes" or "living animalcules in human semen … less than a millionth the size of a coarse grain of sand and with thin, undulating transparent tails". He draws the conclusion that the tails must be operated by means of muscles, tendons and joints (Mol, 2006; Kremer, 1979). van Leeuwenhoek did not study Latin, the scientific language of the day. Nevertheless, his paper amazed and perhaps amused the reigning King of England.

More than 100 years later, in 1784, the first artificial insemination in a dog was reported by the scientist **Lazzaro Spallanzani** (Italian physiologist, 1729-1799). This insemination resulted in the birth of three puppy's 62 days later (Belonoschkin, 1956; Zorgniotti, 1975). It is believed that Spallanzani was the first to report the effects of cooling on human sperm when he noted, in 1776, that sperm cooled by snow became motionless.

The first documented application of artificial insemination in human was done in London in the 1770s by **John Hunter**, which has been called in medical history the "the founder of scientific surgery". A cloth merchant with severe hypospadias was advised to collect the semen (which escaped during coitus) in a warmed syringe and inject the sample into the vagina.

J Marion Sims reported his findings of post-coital tests and 55 inseminations in the mid 1800s. Only one pregnancy occurred but this could be explained by the fact that he believed that ovulation occurred during menstruation. JM Simms was born in Lancaster County (USA) in 1813. In 1863 he began writing his innovative work Clinical Notes on Uterine Surgery, which was controversial but widely read. Its revolutionary approach to female diseases was refreshing and its emphasis on treatment of sterility, including artificial insemination, was ahead of its time.

In 1897 **Heape**, an outstanding reproductive biologist from Cambridge, reported the use of AI in rabbits, dogs and horses. Heape also studied the relationship between seasonality and reproduction, as a result of his research Cambridge became a world centre for reproductive studies.

In 1899 the first attempts to develop practical methods for artificial insemination were described by Ilya Ivanovich Ivanoff (Russia, 1870-1932). Although Ivanoff studied artificial insemination in domestic farm animals, dogs, rabbits and poultry, he was the first to develop methods as we know today in human medicine. He was a pioneer in the selection of superior stallions multiplying their progeny through AI. The work of Ivanoff was taken over by Milovanov, another Russian scientist. He published his paper on "Artificial insemination in Russia" in the Journal of Heredity in 1938. Milovanov established major projects for cattle breeding and designed the first artificial vaginas, very similar to those used today.

The innovating work in Russia inspired Eduard Sörensen from Denmark to organize the first cooperative dairy AI organization in Denmark in 1933, followed by the introduction of the first AI cooperative in the US in 1938 by EJ Perry, a dairyman from New Jersey. In the US and other Western countries the number of AI cooperatives increased rapidly. Nowadays more than 90 % of dairy cows are artificially inseminated in the Netherlands, Denmark and the United Kingdom. November 1, 1939, the first animal, a rabbit, conceived by artificial insemination was exhibited in the United States at the 12th Annual Graduate Fortnight at the New York Academy of Medicine. Gregory Pincus, an American biologist, removed an egg from the ovary of a female rabbit and fertilized it with a salt solution. The egg was then transferred to the uterus of a second rabbit, which functioned as an incubator. Dr. Pincus conducted his experiments at Harvard University.

Considering humans, only after the introduction and availability of donor sperm, artificial insemination became very popular (AID). For many years homologous artificial inseminations were only indicated in cases of physiologic and psychological dysfunction, such as retrograde ejaculation, vaginismus, hypospadias and impotence.

With the routine use of post-coital tests other indications were added such as hostile cervical mucus and immunologic causes with the presence of antispermatozoal antibodies in the cervical mucus.

The first reports on human artificial insemination originated from Guttmacher (1943), Stoughton (1948) and Kohlberg (1953a; 1953b). It was the real start of a new era in assisted reproduction.

Other important research discoveries in animal studies undoubtly influenced the development of artificial insemination, also in human. Phillips and Lardy (1939) were the first to use egg yolk to protect bull sperm cells from temperature shock upon cooling. This protection was explained by the effect of phospholipids and lipoproteins in the egg yolk. Salisbury et al. (1941) improved the media by using egg yolk with sodium citrate, permitting the use of semen at 5° C for up to three days. Polge and co-workers (1949) were the first to freeze fowl and bull spermatozoa by using glycerol in the extender media. In 1950 Cornell University scientists (New York) discovered the benefit of antibiotics added to the sperm solution in artificial insemination processes. The so-called Cornell extender (Foote and Bratton, 1950) contained the antibiotic mixture of penicillin, streptomycin and polymyxim B and was used for many years as the standard. Antibiotics are still used for the protection against possible contamination.

In 1953 Dr. Jerome K. Sherman, an American pioneer in sperm freezing, introduced a simple method of preserving human sperm using glycerol. He combined this with a slow cooling of sperm, and storage with solid carbon dioxide as a refrigerant. Sherman also demonstrated for the first time that frozen sperm, when thawed, were able to fertilize an egg and induce its normal development.

As a result of this research, the first successful human pregnancy with frozen spermatozoa was reported in 1953. Considering the hostile climate for DI at the time (the Cook County Supreme Court ruled that artificial insemination with donor semen was contrary to public policy and good morals) it is not surprising that nearly a decade passed before the first successful birth from frozen sperm was announced in public, a major breakthrough in history.

Considering all these new developments, it could be expected that in the 1970s the sperm bank industry became very popular and commercialized, especially in the United States.

1.3 THE IVF REVOLUTION

The main reason for the renewed interest in artificial insemination in human was undoubtly the introduction of in-vitro fertilisation (IVF) in 1978 by Steptoe and Edwards. In the early days the ejaculate of the husband was inseminated intrauterine without preparation resulting in uterine cramps and increasing the probability of tubal infections. With the arrival of IVF, semen preparation techniques were developed and IUI regained its popularity, being more safe and painless.

These washing procedures are necessary to remove prostaglandins, infectious agents and antigenic proteins. Another substantial advantage of these techniques is the removal of nonmotile spermatozoa, either leucocytes or immature germ cells. This may be an important factor in enhancing sperm quality by a decreased release of lymphokines and/or cytokines and a reduction in the formation of free oxygen radicals after sperm preparation. Sperm preparation techniques should isolate and select sperm cells with intact functional and genetic properties, including normal morphology, minimal DNA damage, and intact cell membranes with functional binding properties.

The final result is a better sperm fertilising ability in vitro and in vivo (Aitken and Clarkson, 1987) and an increasing number of motile sperm that are morphologically normal at the site of fertilization. Bypassing the cervix, which acts as a reservoir for sperm, increases the importance of adequate timing of the insemination.

Most popular are the swim-up procedure, the discontinuous Percoll gradient method, the mini-Percoll (small volume) gradient technique and the use of Sephadex columns.

Novel sperm selection methods (based on sperm surface charge or nonapoptotic sperm selection) show promising results. However, they have not yet established themselves in routine practice, and their purpose for AIH is unknown; more evidence is needed.

Most important milestones in the history of artificial insemination.

1.4 LEGAL, SOCIO-CULTURAL AND RELIGIOUS CONSIDERATIONS SURROUNDING ARTIFICIAL DONOR

Year	Person	Milestone
1677	• Van Leeuwenhoek Antoni	first picture of sperm cells
1780	• Spallanzani Lazzaro	first insemination (in a dog)
1790	• Hunter John	first vaginal insemination in human
1900	• Ivanov Ilya	development of semen extenders
1939	• Pincus Gregory	first animal (rabbit) conceived by artificial insemination
1939	• Phillips & Lardy	egg yolk to protect bull sperm upon cooling
1949	• Polge et al	glycerol in the medium for freezing
1950	• Foote and Bratton	antibiotics in medium
1953	• Sherman Jerome	first pregnancy after AI with frozen sperm
1978	• Steptoe and Edwards	first IVF birth – refinement of semen processing techniques

INSEMINATION

⊙ The moral and social implications of artificial insemination were debated in both the medical and popular press in the United States since 1909, in Europe the debate started in the 1940s. The Catholic Church objected to all forms of artificial insemination, saying that it promoted the vice of onanism and ignored the religious importance of coitus. The main criticism was that artificial insemination with donor semen was a form of adultery promoting the vice of masturbation. Other critics were concerned that AID could encourage eugenic government policies.

⊙ Nevertheless, the demand for donor sperm increased tremendously. After the first successful pregnancy from frozen sperm, reported in 1953, the development of a thriving sperm-bank industry starting in the 1970s and the commercialization of AID became unavoidable. The growing number of AID's raised new concerns leading to new regulations. Because of the possible transmission of sexually transmitted diseases, including HIV, when using fresh sperm screening for infections of donors became mandatory. The use of fresh donor semen samples almost disappeared.

⦿ Another concern is the possibility to donate semen many times. In order to diminish the chances of unknowing marriage of biological siblings among AID children some government regulations tightly restrict the number of times a single donor's semen may be used and/or restrict the number of children by a given donor.

⦿ Sociocultural concerns with biological paternity and the maintenance of the heterosexual, married couple as the basis of the family remain important in many countries. A lot of countries all over the world have not approved the use of AI with donor semen for single women and lesbian couples yet. Another point of debate is whether the donor has to be anonymous or non-anonymous, and when to inform and what to tell AID children about their biological parentage, if non-anonymous donors are used. Is it possible and/or advisable to use sperm of relatives, such as brothers or the father? Whether or not to pay the donors and sexing of sperm by DNA quantification using flow cytometry instrumentation became a point of discussion.

⦿ The historical story of artificial insemination is a successful one; the worldwide acceptance of artificial insemination in animals provided the impetus for the innovation and development of many technologies which we are nowadays familiar with such as gamete cryopreservation, ovarian stimulation and cycle regulation, embryo freezing and cloning. Many of the principles nowadays used in human artificial insemination are adapted from domestic animal studies, especially from cattle. The use of frozen/thawed donor samples and the renewed interest in sperm washing procedures due to the introduction of IVF were the most important milestones in the history of human artificial insemination.

⦿ Intrauterine insemination with husband's sperm turned out to be a valuable first choice treatment before starting more invasive and more expensive techniques of assisted reproduction for many subfertile patients.

⦿ The increasing demand of lesbians and single women for AI with donor semen is another challenge in many countries worldwide. Many debates, socio-cultural and ethical, are to be expected in the near future. The issue of using anonymous and/or non-anonymous donors will be one of them.

1.5 ADVANTAGES OF ARTIFICIAL INSEMINATION OVER NATURAL SERVICE

Artificial insemination (AI) is one of the most efficient tools accessible to dairy farmers to improve productivity and profitability of dairy enterprise. In artificial insemination the bulls of superior quality can be efficiently exploited with the least concern for their location in faraway places. There are a lot of advantages of AI over natural services with bulls. They are as follows:

- Boosts efficiency of bull usage: During natural mating, a bull will donate much more semen than is theoretically needed to make a pregnancy. On the other hand, collected semen can be diluted and extended to make hundreds of semen doses from a single ejaculate which can be easily carried one place to another, promoting multiple inseminations in females in different geographical locations and semen can be stored for long periods of time

- Cost Effectiveness: No necessity of maintenance of breeding bulls. Hence, the expenditure on maintenance of breeding bull is saved.

- Checks disease transmission: Natural mating allows the transmission of venereal e.g.,diseases between males and females. On the other hand, for AI, semen is regularly tested for its quality, possible infections hence allows checking of the spread of certain venereal diseases. Contagious abortion, vibriosis.

- Promotes Breeding Efficiency: By routine examination of semen after collection and frequent checking on fertility make early detection of inferior bulls and better breeding efficiency is warranted.

- The progeny testing can be employed at an early age.

- The semen of an elite bull can be used even after the death of that sire.

- It makes possible the mating of animals with great variations in body size with no injury to either of the animal.

- It is useful to inseminate the cows denying to stand or accept the bulls at the time of oestrum.

- Useful in maintaining the perfect breeding and calving records.

- Artificial Insemination enhances the rate of conception.

- Artificial Insemination allows the use of old, heavy and injured sires.

- Artificial Insemination when linked to oestrous synchronization programme, can promote a more consistent, uniform calf crop production.

1.6 SHORTCOMINGS OF ARTIFICIAL INSEMINATION

- ⊙ Dairy farmers have numerous arguments against Artificial Insemination. In general, an AI program would need more intensive management of the herd like a sound nutrition program (cows in good body condition), good record keeping in the farm, an efficient herd health program, precise heat detection and a well-trained AI technician.

- ⊙ Poor management in one or more of these fields might result in poorer success rates. Few major drawbacks of AI are mentioned below:

  i. Requires well-trained personnel and special tools.
  ii. Takes more time than natural services.
  iii. The AI operator needs to have the knowledge of the structure and function of reproduction in the dairy animals.
  iv. Improper cleanliness of instruments and unhygienic conditions may lead to declined conception.
  v. If the bull is not appropriately examined, the spreading of venereal diseases will be increased.

1.7 SEMEN COLLECTION

Semen collection refers to the process of obtaining semen from domestic animals with the use Semen can be collected from animals via three distinct methods/techniques. These involve:

- ⊙ Use of artificial vagina

- ⊙ Rectal massage method

- ⊙ Electro-ejaculation of various methods, for the purpose of artificial insemination or medical study.

The technique used depends on the species and condition of the individual animal concerned.

1.7.1 Artificial Vagina

Several methods of obtaining semen have been developed. Artificial vaginas (AV) are used to collect semen from many species, most prominently cattle and horses, but also sheep, goats, rabbits and even cats. An AV uses thermal and mechanical stimulation to induce ejaculation. An AV is composed of a tube with an outer rubber lining that hold water, into which is placed an inner liner that is lubricated just prior to use. The outer liner is filled and pressurized somewhat with water at 42-48 degrees Celsius.

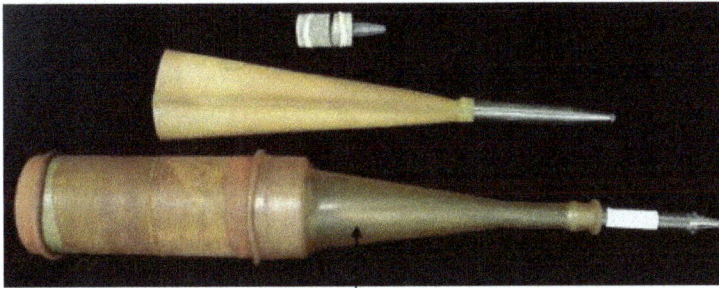

1.7.2 AV Used in Cattle, Dog and Cat

Components Parts of Artificial vagina

Artificial vaginas are of different shapes and sizes. The component parts are listed below:

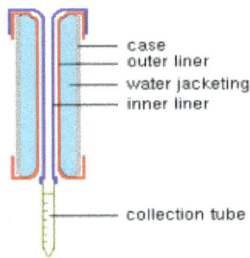

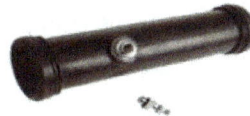

Source: www.innovis.org.uk

    a.   Rigid rubber casing with an opening at both end

    b.   Rough-textured latex inner liner

    c.   Rubber band

    d.   Rubber funnel

    e.   Graduated glass collection tube

    f.   Insulated and zippered jacket during cold season

1.7.3 Facilities Needed For Semen Collection

There are some key facilities that must be put in place for effective semen collection to be realised. Some of these facilities are listed below:

- Facilities for safety of collector
- Earthen floor to prevent slipping
- Means to restrain teaser animals
- Easy access for semen collection

1.7.4 Materials Needed For Semen Collection

There are some essential materials that are needed for effective semen collection, especially when artificial vagina is the preferred method of collection. Some of these materials are listed as follow:

- Artificial vagina
- Lubricant (sterile)
- Glass rod
- Collection tube
- Hot water at required temperature

After semen collection exercise, it becomes necessary that artificial vagina and other materials used be cleaned, sterilized and stored properly. The inner liner and rubber funnel should be soaked for 5 min. in 70% ethanol after washing, and then dried under UV light in a dust-free cabinet.

1.7.5 Sexual Stimulation Prior to Collection with the Artificial Vagina

There is need for sexual stimulation of animal in semen collection. This will influence positively the volume of ejaculate from such animal. The effects of such stimulations are not well defined in boar and stallion, but notable in bull .The main reasons for sexual stimulation are:

- To ensure that bull will mount and ejaculate reasonably, and
- To ensure that collection of maximum number of sperm with highest possible quality per ejaculate are realized

1.7.5.1 Steps Involved in Sexual Stimulation

- By exposing bulls to teaser for several min. or 2 to 3 false mounting
- Introducing a new teaser animal
- Moving teaser animal to different area
- Presenting 2 teasers
- Allowing teaser or another bull to mount the bull to be collected
- Bringing new bull into the collection area

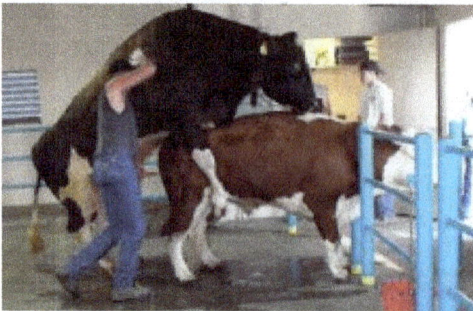

Fig. 1 A Faulse mounting

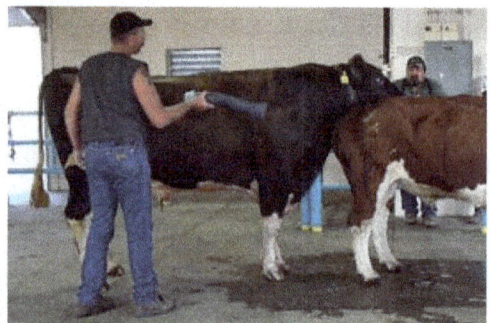

Fig. 1: B Sustained errection

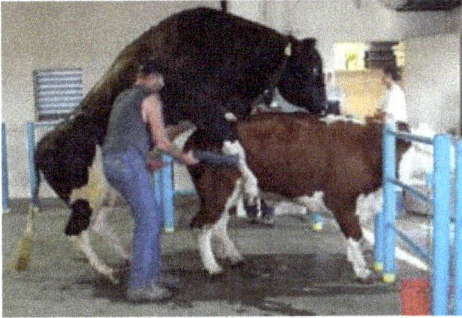

| Fig. 1: C Collector ready with AV | Fig. 1: D Diversion of penis into AV |

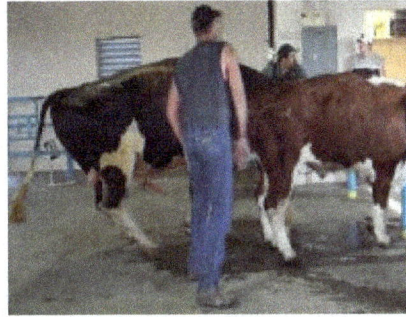

Source: *http://www.vivo.colostate.edu/hbooks/pathphys/reprod/semeneval/bull.html*

1.7.5.2 Rectal Massage

Rectal massage is the stimulation of the animal by massaging the vesicular gland and ampullae by way of rectum for semen collection. These organs take part in the sexual response cycle, and are essential for ejaculation. These organs are found to be most active during time of ejaculation. Due to close proximity to the anterior rectal wall, it can be stimulated manually via the anus. It should be noted that rectal massage method is the most appropriate way for semen collection in cock apart from other ruminants.

1.7.5.3 Electro-Ejaculation

Electro-ejaculation involves applying a series of short, low-voltage pulses of current to the pelvic nerves which are involved in the ejaculatory response. It sounds like an extremely unpleasant experience, but doesn't seem to cause much distress in bulls (although they do need to be securely restrained), and is conducted under anesthesia in many species.

With few exceptions, electro-ejaculation is the only technique useful for collecting semen from wild animals, in which case the male is anesthetized prior to the procedure. Another advantage of electro-ejaculation is that it does not require a mount animal, and can be applied in the field using a battery-powered unit. Finally, electro-ejaculation can be used to obtain semen from animals that are physically incapable of mounting due to musculoskeletal disease or injury. It is used for collecting semen from animal that cannot mount due to spinal cord injury.

With bulls, where there is abundant experience collecting semen by both artificial vagina and electro-ejaculation, the samples collected using an electro-ejaculator usually have a larger volume (due to excessive accessory gland secretion) and a lower number of sperm. Three pieces of equipment are required for electro-ejaculation. The electro-ejaculator itself is a power supply with rheostats to control the amplitude of the delivered current and lots of circuitry to prevent accidental electrocution. Second, one needs a collection tube, usually attached to a latex rubber cone ("loving cup") in which to collect the semen. Finally, the pulses of current are applied through an electro-ejaculator probe.

The probe is inserted into the rectum such that the electrodes lie within the pelvic cavity. Older probes had circular electrodes, which often caused undesirable muscle contractions; probes with parallel electrodes on one side minimize this problem. Successful electro-ejaculation of an animal demands skill. It is not simply a matter of punching buttons and turning knobs, but requires finesse in determining the proper timing and amplitude of pulses to apply to a given male

Below are the diagrams of different types of electro-ejaculator used in different species ranging from small to large.

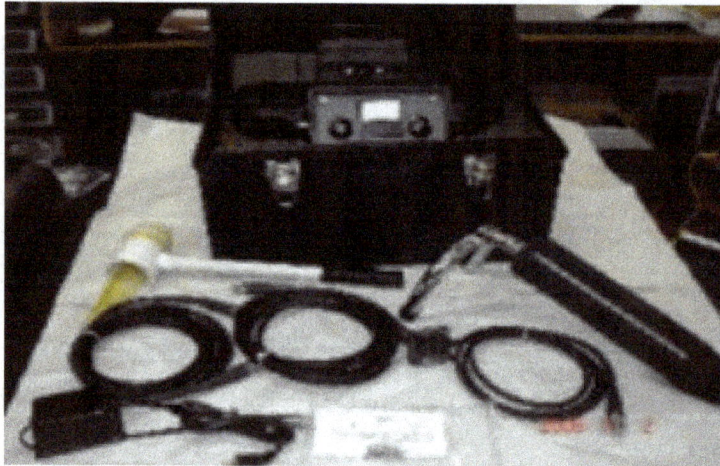

Fig. 2: Electroejaculator

Source: *http://www.allvet.org/electroejac.htm*

Conditions applicable to the collection of semen

- ◉ The floor of the mounting area should be clean and provide safe footing. A dusty floor should be avoided.

- ◉ The hindquarters of the teaser, whether a dummy or a live teaser animal, should be kept clean. A dummy should be cleaned completely after each period of collection. A teaser animal should have its hindquarters cleaned carefully before each collecting session. The dummy or hindquarters of the teaser animals should be sanitized after the collection of each ejaculate. Disposable plastic covers may be used.

- ◉ The hand of the person collecting the semen should not come into contact with the animal's penis. Disposable gloves should be worn by the collector and changed for each collection.

- ◉ The artificial vagina should be cleaned completely after each collection where relevant. It should be dismantled, it's various parts washed, rinsed and dried, and kept protected from dust. The inside of the body of the device and the cone should be disinfected before re- assembly using approved disinfection techniques such as those involving the use of alcohol, ethylene oxide or steam. Once re-assembled, it should be kept in a cupboard which is regularly cleaned and disinfected.

- The lubricant used should be clean. The rod used to spread the lubricant should be clean and should not be exposed to dust between successive collections.

- The artificial vagina should not be shaken after ejaculation, otherwise lubricant and debris may pass down the cone to join the contents of the collecting tube.

- When successive ejaculates are being collected, a new artificial vagina should be used for each mounting. The vagina should also be changed when the animal has inserted its penis without ejaculating.

- The collecting tubes should be sterile, and either disposable or sterilised by autoclaving or heating in an oven at 180°C for at least 30 minutes. They should be kept sealed to prevent exposure to the environment while awaiting use.

- After semen collection, the tube should be left attached to the cone and within its sleeve until it has been removed from the collection room for transfer to the laboratory

2

ANATOMY OF THE REPRODUCTIVE TRACTS

2.1 INTRODUCTION: AN OVERVIEW

The reproductive system has multiple functions in animals. The most important one is the production of gametes, haploid cells specialized in the transmission of the genetic information. Male gametes are the spermatozoids and female gametes are the oocytes. The fusion of one spermatozoid and one oocyte results in a diploid cell known as zygote. One zygote divides and gives rise many cell lineages that after differentiation form a complete new organism.

The reproductive system is morphologically different in males compared to females. The differences arise very early during the embryo development. Building male or female reproductive structures will later determine the morphological features of the adult animal, mainly the sexual secondary features like muscle development, bone structures, body hair, mammilar structures, fat distribution, behavior, etcetera. This is the so-called sexual dimorphism. Being a male or a female is mostly determined by sexual chromosomes. In humans, XX sexual chromosomes give female morphology and XY chromosomes give male morphology. However, in other vertebrates, like reptiles and fish, environment variables, like temperature, may determine the sex of the animal. Some fish species may behave as hermaphrodites, so that they can produce male and female gametes.

Successful artificial insemination depends on the understanding of the organs involved in reproduction, in order to know where to deposit semen for optimal conception rates.

2.2 FEMALE REPRODUCTIVE TRACT

The vulva is the visible exterior segment of the reproductive tract, located beneath the tail and immediately below the anus. It consists of two vertical lips or labia. It is the entry to the female reproductive tract during copulation.

Apposition of the moist vulva lips together with its sphincter form a physical barrier that prevents entry of foreign material and contamination of the female reproductive tract. When the doe is on heat the vulva may be swollen, reddened and mucus may be seen coming through the lips.

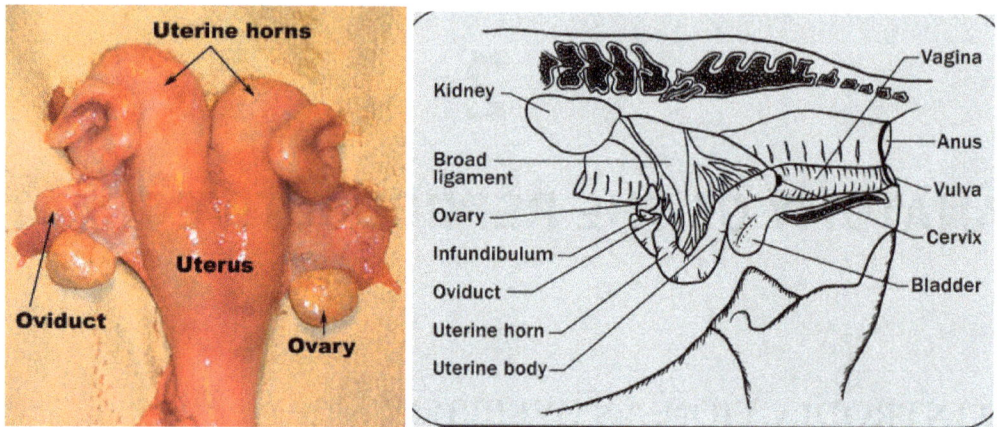

Fig. 1: Structure of the female reproductive tract.

Anterior to the vulva is the vestibule, at the base of which is the clitoris and urethra where urine exits through. During AI one has to be careful not to introduce the AI pipette into the urethra. The vagina is directly in front of the vestibule. It is a tubular structure and is the organ of copulation where the buck deposits semen during mating.

Cranial to the vagina is the cervix. Compared to the rest of tubular genitalia, it is a firm structure and forms the joint between the vagina and the uterus. It is about one to one-half inches long, contains about five cervical rings or folds, and is referred to as the neck of the uterus. It is usually closed to create a physical barrier that prevents foreign objects from entering the uterus. During pregnancy, a thick mucus plug closes the cervix to keep out material from entering the uterus and thus safeguarding the pregnancy. When the doe is on heat the cervix opens and secretes mucus to allow for movement of spermatozoa to the site of fertilization. This opening of the cervix during oestrus is the one that allows passage of the insemination pipette through the cervix in order to perform AI. At the end of pregnancy the cervix will fully open to allow for delivery of the kid.

After the cervix comes the uterus. It consists of a small uterine body and two separate horns (cornua). It is the organ that houses the growing fetus during pregnancy and also produces substances (hormones) that are involved in the regulation of the reproductive cycle.

Oviducts project from the front end of each uterine horn. Each oviduct is a thin tubular structure and is a conduit between its ovary and uterine horn. The oviduct is the place where fertilization takes place. At its tip, the oviduct opens like a funnel (infundibulum) near the ovary. The infundibulum is the structure that receives the ova released from the ovary, directs them to the opening of the oviduct for transport to the site of fertilization.

The ovaries are the innermost structures of the reproductive tract. They produce the egg (ovum), and also the hormones that are responsible for oestrus and maintaining pregnancy. From puberty on throughout the reproductive life, the ovary contains follicles (fluid filled structures in which the ovum develops and is suspended) and a corpus luteum (a temporary structure formed by a ruptured mature follicle that has released its ovum). The fluid inside the follicle is rich in the hormone estrogen. At a particular time, the follicle ruptures to produce the egg, in a process referred to as ovulation. After the follicle has ruptured and released the egg, a yellow body, the corpus luteum, develops at the site of the ruptured follicle. It is a structure that grows rapidly on the ovary and then undergoes lysis (death) after some days if the doe does not get pregnant. The corpus luteum produces the hormone progesterone, which regulates the oestrus cycle and is also responsible for maintenance of pregnancy.

2.3 MALE REPRODUCTIVE TRACT

Visible parts of the male reproductive tract are scrotum, prepuce and penis. The scrotum is the muscular sac hanging between the hind legs and it contains the testes, which are the paired male gonads. The scrotum supports and protects the testes and plays a major role in temperature regulation. It maintains the temperature of the testes at 3 to 5°C below body temperature for optimal functioning of the testes. The testes produce the male gametes (spermatozoa) and secrete the male sex hormone, testosterone. Testosterone is required for the development of the male sexual characteristics, maintenance of normal sexual behavior and sperm production. The penis is the organ of copulation which allows the buck to deposit semen into the vagina of the doe. At the tip of the penis is a thin tubular structure, the urethral process, which sprays the semen in and around the cervix of the doe. The penis is covered by the prepuce, a fold of skin which protects it.

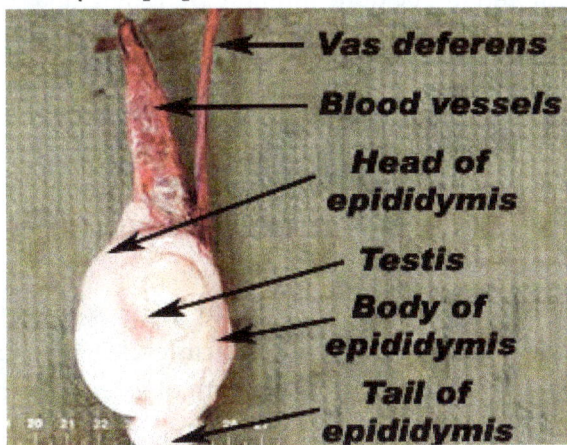

Fig: 2: Abattoir specimen showing parts of the buck's reproductive system.

The other parts of the male reproductive tract are the accessory glands, which are not externally visible. They are the seminal vesicles, prostate, bulbourethral glands and ampulla. They add fluid to the sperm, together forming semen, which is the one produced by the buck during mating in a process referred to as ejaculation. These fluids contain sugars which nourish the sperm, provide buffers hence prevent rapid changes in pH, and other chemicals that protect and propel the sperm through the male reproductive tract during ejaculation. The vas deferens is the duct through which sperm moves from the testes to the urethra. The amount of sperm in an ejaculate and the volume of the ejaculate depend on the season, age of the buck, level of sexual activity, breed and the individual buck itself. A normal range of ejaculate volume in the buck is 0.5 to 1.5 ml, containing 1.5 to 5 billion sperm per ml of ejaculate.

- ◉ As part of the practical session for the above, female and male reproductive organs in live animals and abattoirs specimens are examined and used to illustrate or explain the functional anatomy of the different parts of the reproductive system.

2.4 FEMALE REPRODUCTIVE CYCLE

Young female goats or doelings reach puberty at about 6 to 8 months of age and may be bred at 7 to 10 months of age depending on how they have been fed and grown. Puberty is the stage of sexual development at which the doe is capable of getting pregnant, if it is mated. Various factors affect the onset of puberty, including, healthcare, nutrition, season of birth and breed. Poor nutrition delays puberty; smaller breeds of goats attain puberty earlier; whereas kids born during the season when feed is plenty and of good quality attain puberty earlier. Breeding of does for the first time should be based on body weight as proportion of mature weight, and not age at which puberty is attained. It is recommended that young females should be bred after they have attained 60 to 70% of their adult weight to ensure kidding ease and avoid dystocia. Puberty is more dependent on body weight than age, so breeding should not be done until the right weight is attained.

2.5 THE OESTRUS CYCLE

Once puberty is attained, the doe comes on heat (oestrus) at regular intervals thereafter. Oestrus is associated with the desire to be bred. This behavior (oestrus) is repeated at regular intervals, unless interrupted by pregnancy or disease, and this repetition is referred to as the oestruscycle. Therefore, the oestruscycle is defined as the number of days between two consecutive periods of oestrus.

A healthy doe will come into oestrus every 20 to 21 days, except when pregnant. In different individuals and breeds, however, the oestrus cycle length can range between 17 to 25 days. To help determine the estruscycle length of each breeding doe, the producer should maintain a breeding diary or records. Good records are important for informing a breeding program, as they can help the breeder predict when a doe is likely to come on heat, and thus enable more careful observation for heat signs at that time. Additionally, good records will help determine if a doe has a problem, if she comes on heat too early, delays, or fails to come on heat at the expected time and she has not been previously bred.

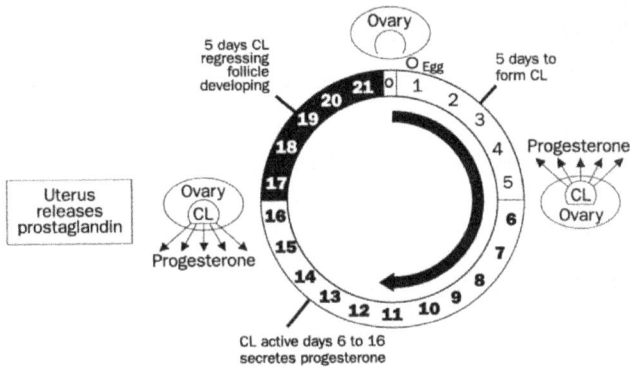

Fig. 3: Schematic representation of the oestruscycle.

When does are on heat, they exhibit various physiological and behavioral changes, referred to as signs of oestrus.

These signs of heat are:

◉ Bleating continuously

◉ The vulva may become swollen, reddened and may appear moist, dirty or muddy due to mucus discharge from the reproductive tract

◉ There is frequent twitching of the tail

◉ She may urinate small amounts of urine frequently

◉ A clear, stringy mucus discharge may be seen from the vulva (may mat hair in perineal area)

◉ The doe displays restlessness

◉ She may mount other goats and stand to be mounted

The doe may not exhibit all the above signs, and under adverse conditions, such as extreme heat and injuries, may not show any signs at all. Standing to be mounted is the most obvious or accurate sign that a doe is on heat. Standing to be mounted will be enhanced in the presence of a buck. Does not in oestrus will always resist mounting attempts by the buck or other does. Standing oestrus in does may last for 12 to 36 hours.

2.6 HORMONAL CONTROL OF THE OESTRUS CYCLE

Upon reaching puberty, every three weeks the doe's brain signals the follicle in the ovary to start developing the egg. The signal from the brain is from the hypothalamus which releases the hormone Gonadotropin Releasing hormone, or GnRH. This hormone stimulates the pituitary gland at the base of the brain to produce gonadotropin hormones, Follicle Stimulating Hormone (FSH) and Luteinizing Hormone (LH). Follicle stimulating hormone, as the name implies, initiates the development of follicles on the ovary from small pinhead sized structures to fluid-filled structures that are about half an inch in diameter. As a follicle grows in size, fluid accumulates in its cavity and secretes estrogen hormone. Estrogen is the female sex hormone. It is secreted into the blood stream and circulates throughout the body. Estrogen production is greatest when the follicle reaches its maximum size. High levels of estrogen act on the does' brain resulting in the changes in the doe that are manifested as heat signs. It affects the nervous system causing behavioral changes such as restlessness, increased vocalization, twitching of the tail, lack of appetite, desire to mate by standing to be mounted, and also affects the reproductive system by increasing blood flow to the reproductive tract causing swelling of the vulva, reddening of the vulva, and the mucus discharge seen from the vulva during oestrus.

Once estrogen levels from the mature follicle reach a certain threshold, they stimulate a peak release of LH (LH surge). The LH surge causes the mature follicle to undergo changes that result into its rupture and release of the egg. This rupture of the mature follicle and release of the egg is referred to as ovulation. After ovulation, the cells inside the ruptured follicle begin to grow and undergo changes (luteinization) under the influence of the gonadotropin hormone LH to form a gland called the Corpus Luteum (CL), the yellow body. The CL produces progesterone, the hormone of pregnancy. Its function is to prepare the uterus for accepting the fertilized egg, and to maintain pregnancy by preventing recurrence of the oestruscycle during gestation. If fertilization does not occur, the CL is destroyed at about 16 days after heat and consequently stops producing progesterone. Destruction of the CL is caused by the hormone prostaglandin F2α (PGF2α) which is produced by the inner wall of the uterus. The drop in progesterone concentration is consequently followed by a rise in gonadotropin release (FSH and LH), development of another follicle(s) and egg(s), and recurrence of heat about 20 to 21 days after the previous heat period. This cycle will continue throughout the reproductive life of the doe and will only be interrupted by pregnancy, disease, malnutrition or senility.

When the egg is fertilized and accepted, the presence of the developing foetus in the uterus sends a signal to the dam causing the CL to remain active and produce progesterone for maintenance of pregnancy. This process is referred to as maternal recognition of pregnancy.

2.7 HEAT DETECTION

Heat detection is one of the factors that greatly determines the success or failure of any AI program. Under natural mating conditions, the buck accurately picks the does that are on heat, and if he is normal, promptly mates them.

However, with AI, the inseminator replaces the buck. Therefore, for optimal conception rates to be achieved with AI, the doe has to be inseminated at the appropriate time, and thus it is important to recognize when a doe is on heat and to breed her at the right time. For a successful genetic improvement program and efficient delivery of superior genetics through AI service, good heat detection is therefore critical. It is recommended that a person be designated to observe animals in the herd for heat signs at least twice a day.

Sufficient time (at least 15 minutes depending on herd size) should be allocated for the exercise, and it should not coincide with periods of activities, such as feeding, that would distract the attention of the animals. Preferably it should be done during the cooler parts of the day (morning and evening) when the animals are resting. Accurate heat detection greatly enhances the success of an AI program.

2.8 OESTRUS DETECTION TECHNIQUES

- ◉ Having a buck in close proximity to the does. Does in heat are more easily identifiable if a buck is housed nearby.

- ◉ The signs of heat will be more intense, and she will pace restlessly along the pen in an effort to try and get to the buck or she will stand close to the fence with the hope of enticing the buck.

- ◉ Time to observe heat. Animals tend to be more sexually active during the cooler parts of the day (around dawn and dusk) and this is a good time to observe for heat. Thirty minutes before morning feeding/milking and 30 minutes after evening feeding/milking should be used for heat detection. Putting a number of does together in one area or pen will facilitate the interaction between animals and make it easier to notice the heat signs.

- ◉ Using a teaser buck. This is a buck that has been prepared in various ways so that he can be able to pick out does that are on heat but cannot be able to make them pregnant. A teaser buck could be an entire buck with an apron or whole penis has been deviated, hence is able to detect and mount does on heat but whose penis will be unable to enter the female genitalia; it could also be a vasectomized buck, who will detect does on heat, mount and copulate with them but is incapable of depositing spermatozoa into the female reproductive system.

- ◉ Using a teaser with a marking harness. Markers will leave identifications on the ramps of does that stood to be mounted (were on heat). This way labor is saved as someone does not have to be with the herd to check for the does standing to be mounted. The marked does would be noted in the morning or evening each day.

- ◉ Anticipate heat with records. Using well-kept reproductive records, it is possible to predict when the doe would come on heat, thus enabling closer observation.

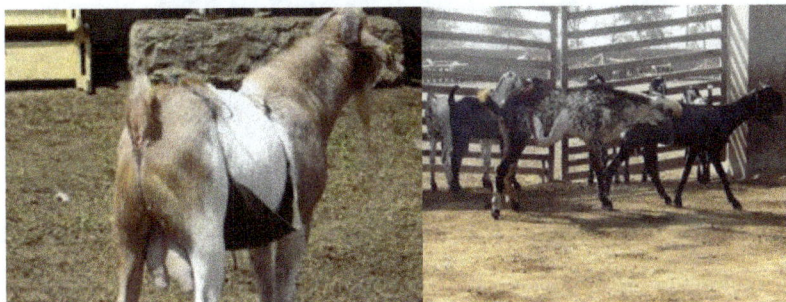

Fig. 4: A buck for heat detection with an apron.

2.9 TROUBLE-SHOOTING HEAT DETECTION

2.9.1 Semen Storage

Semen to be used for AI is collected from selected bucks, processed and safely stored. The processing includes dilution of the ejaculate with a semen extender in order to produce many doses from a given ejaculate. Cryoprotectant are added to protect the spermatozoa from being destroyed during the freezing process. The extended semen is then packed in labelled straws and stored frozen in liquid nitrogen in tanks at -196°C. At this temperature, the spermatozoa remain inactive but viable. Each semen straw contains the necessary number of spermatozoa for one insemination to be able to cause conception. The straw is labelled with information regarding the buck from which it was collected (sire code and breed), date of processing and semen processing station code.

Liquid nitrogen tanks (Figures 5, 6 and 7) are large metal vacuum containers used to store frozen semen. They come in different sizes and can store up to 100,000 semen straws for many years. The tanks are well insulated to help maintain temperatures at -196° C which is necessary for the semen to remain viable. At this low temperature, the metabolism of the sperm cells is stopped and they remain in resting state. The working parts of the tank are a lid, styrofoam cork, canisters, canes, the inner chamber that holds the liquid nitrogen, and a spider to keep the canisters from moving around. The cork is 4-6 inches in length with grooves on the sides for the canister handles. The cork fits loosely in the neck of the tank, allowing for the evaporating nitrogen gas to escape. If capped too tightly, the gas would build up pressure in the tank resulting in an explosion.

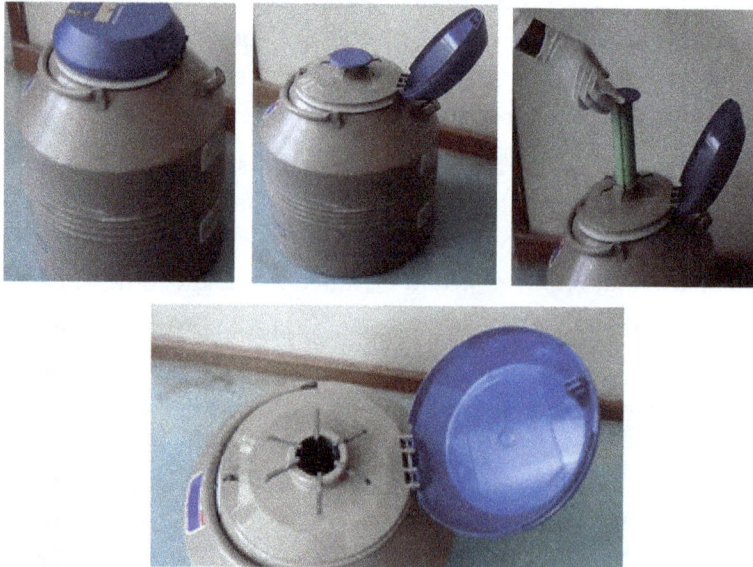

Fig. 5: Liquid nitrogen tank (left), with lid open (center), showing grooved Styrofoam cork (right).

Canisters hang from the top of the tank supported by their wire handles which protrude to the outside at the top of the tank. The canisters are usually six in number and their long wire handles are used to lift the cylindrical end of the canister in and out of the tank. The canisters hold the canes that contain the semen straws. For ease of management of the semen inventory, the canister handle and/or the groove that supports it on the tank are numbered to facilitate quick identification of the semen straw that needs to be picked from the tank.

Great care should be taken when handling a liquid nitrogen tank and its contents. Close attention should be paid to the vacuum port. Liquid nitrogen should not be spilt on it or loss of vacuum may occur rendering the tank dysfunctional. Signs of vacuum loss include a strong hissing sound and ice crystal formation around the neck of the tank. It is important to monitor liquid nitrogen levels on a regular basis to make sure the levels are adequate in order to avoid semen damage. A liquid nitrogen tank measuring stick should be used for estimating the liquid nitrogen levels.

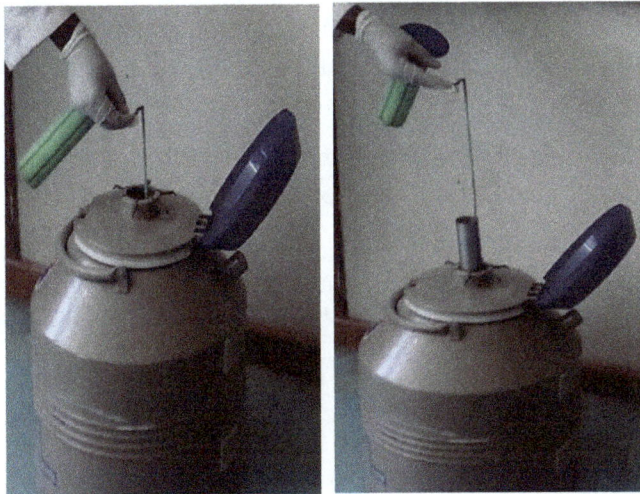

Fig. 6: Wire handle raising the canister from the liquid nitrogen tank.

2.9.2 It is Important to Take Good Care of the Tank

Regularly replenish the liquid nitrogen in the tank to avoid levels falling low and damaging the semen. Liquid nitrogen is lost through evaporation, and each time the tank is opened. If the semen straw is not submerged in the liquid nitrogen its temperature will rise resulting in death of the spermatozoa.

- ◉ Canisters should not be raised more than 25cm above the neck of the tank, to prevent semen straws from being exposed to high temperatures as this may damage the spermatozoa. Once raised, the canister should be lowered back into the tank as soon as possible, preferably, within 3 seconds. This avoids excessive temperature fluctuation within the semen straws. When a canister is raised and then lowered into the tank, a bubbling/boiling sound is heard. This is due to the temperature change resulting from the relatively warmer canister heating up the liquid nitrogen.

- ⦿ A semen inventory should be maintained to track semen straw quantities, use, replacement and their canister assignment.

- ⦿ This allows quick and easy location of the desired semen straw when it is needed for insemination.

- ⦿ The top of each cane should be marked, clearly identifying the cane's contents. If possible, avoid storing semen straws from more than one buck in a single cane.

- ⦿ A catalog or map of the tank's contents should be maintained. Any change in inventory within the tank should be noted in the map.

- ⦿ The stopper should never be forced into the tank. Doing so will damage the tank, reducing its longevity.

- ⦿ Dents to the tank should be avoided. Dents reduce the total volume of the tank and hence the liquid nitrogen holding time. Such tanks will require more frequent replenishment with liquid nitrogen, increasing the maintenance costs of the tank. Tanks should not be set unprotected on gravel, dirt, or concrete.

- ⦿ They should be stored unboxed, in a clean, dry, visible, secure area, on surfaces such as clean carpet, wood, cardboard, a rubber mat, to protect the bottom from dents and scratches.

- ⦿ The tank should be kept clean and hygienic to avoid contaminating semen strawsduring AI and also the likelihood of spreading disease from one farm to the next.

3

FIXED TIME AI PROTOCOLS: A TOOL FOR EFFECTIVE REPRODUCTIVE MANAGEMENT OF DAIRY ANIMALS

3.1 INTRODUCTION: AN OVERVIEW

- Estrus synchronization is one of the most important and widely applicable reproductive biotechnologies available for cattle. The major factor limiting optimum reproductive performance on many cattle farms is failure to detect cows in heat in a timely and accurate manner.

- Poor estrus detection results in excessive number of days open which causes long calving intervals and economic losses to the farmers. A study conducted to evaluate efficiency of visual estrus detection showed that only 56% of cows observed twice a day for 30 minutes could be detected in standing estrus as compared to 95% of cows detected following 24 hours a day visual monitoring. This shows that estrus detection is time consuming and labour intensive process.

- Estrus synchronizing is an effective way to minimize the time and labour required to detect standing estrus for artificial insemination. In addition, some estrus synchronization protocols (progestin-based protocols) can induce a proportion of anestrous cows to begin estrous cycles providing more chances for cows to conceive during a defined breeding season.

3.2 ESTRUS SYNCHRONIZATION

- Estrus synchronization is the manipulation of the reproductive process i.e. estrous cycle so that a group of females exhibit standing estrus and can be bred with normal fertility during a short, predefined time interval.

- This control facilitates breeding in two important ways i.e. it reduces and in some cases eliminates the labour of detecting estrus (heat), and it allows the farmers to schedule the breeding.

3.2.1 Basic Approach for Estrus Synchronization

Basic approach is to control the timing of the onset of estrus by controlling the length of the estrous cycle. Two approaches are used for controlling estrous cycle length :

- Shortening of Luteal phase – by administration of Prostaglandin (PGF2α) to regress the corpus luteum (CL) before the time of natural luteolysis.

- Prolongation of Luteal phase – by administration of Progesterone or more commonly synthetic progestins to temporarily prolong the luteal phase or delay onset of estrus.

3.2.2 Estrus Synchronization Protocols

- A variety of estrus synchronization protocols are available which involves use of hormones like Prostaglandins, GnRH, Estradiol esters, progesterone or progestagin devices.

- The PGF protocols does not facilitate fixed time insemination whereas, most of the GnRH based and estradiol based protocols facilitate fixed time insemination and are widely used.

3.2.3 Prostaglandins

- Prostaglandin (PGF2α) is a naturally occurring hormone. During the normal estrous cycle of a non-pregnant animal, PGF2α is released from the uterus 16 to 18 days after the animal was in heat. This release of PGF2α functions to destroy the corpus luteum (CL). The CL is a structure in the ovary that produces the hormone progesterone and prevents the animal from returning to estrus. The release of PGF2α from the uterus is the triggering mechanism that results in the animal returning to estrus every 21 days. Commercially available PGF2α (Lutalyse, Estrumate, Clostenol etc.) gives the herd owner the ability to simultaneously remove the CL from all cycling animals at a predetermined time that is convenient for heat detection and breeding.

- The major limitation of PGF2α is that it is not effective on animals that do not possess a CL. This includes animals within 6 to 7 days of a previous heat, prepubertal heifers and postpartum anestrous cows. Despite these limitations, prostaglandins are the simplest method to synchronize estrus in cattle.

3.2.4 Single Shot PGF or 6-Day Heat Detection Plus PGF

- A lower cost alternative is to breed animals to natural heats for 6 days and then inject the unbred animals with PGF2α and breed over the next 5 to 7 days.

This system allows all cycling animals to be bred during a two week period and requires less PGF injections/head. Although this system is conservative in terms of hormone usage, it is probably one of the more labor intensive synchronization options.

- If <20% of the animals have been inseminated following 6 days of heat detection, there may be a cyclicity problem. Don't waste time and money trying to synchronize a herd of cows that are not cycling. Instead, evaluate the body condition score, herd health and nutrition level of the herd.

3.2.5 Two-Shot PGF Protocol

- The most common method of synchronization with PGF2α is to inject all animals and breed those that come into heat over the next 5 to 7 days. Animals not detected is estrus after the first injection are re-injected 14 days later and bred over the next 5 to 7 day period. Animals detected in standing heat should be inseminated 8-12 hours later. If labor availability is a limitation, all heat detection and breeding can be delayed until after the second PGF injection. This allows the producer to breed a high percentage of the herd during a single 5-7 day period, but requires two doses of PGF/head versus 1.3 to 1.5 doses/head if animals are bred after each injection. Overall estrus response rates may be slightly reduced (~5%) when animals are bred only after the second injection as some animals that responded to the first injection may not respond again to the second.

- Although recommendations were to inject PGF2α at 11-day intervals, from a scheduling consideration, the 14-day interval is much easier to implement. The second injection is always 2 weeks down on the calendar from the first and all activities (injections, heat detection, breeding) are conducted on the same days of the week from one week to the next. Animals that respond to the first injection, but are not detected in estrus, will be between day 7 and 9 of the cycle at the next injection using the 11-day interval. These "early" CLs typically do not respond to PGF as well as older more mature ones. Using a 14-day interval, a missed heat from the first injection will be on days 10 to 12 of the cycle at the second injection. This 3-day difference significantly improves the probability of the animal responding again.

3.2.6 PGF Limitations

- Fixed-time AI - Fixed-time insemination after single or double injections of PGF alone seldom yields acceptable results and in general, is not recommended.

- Suckled cows - A major limitation of PGF is that it only works in cycling animals. Therefore, PGF-based protocols work very well in properly managed beef or dairy heifers and in many dairy herd systematic breeding programs. However, even in the best managed herds, some of the suckled cows may still be anestrus at the beginning of the breeding season. In such situations, use of PGF in combination with GnRH and/or a progestin source are much more effective options.

- Estrus and ovulation is highly variable due to differences between cows in the stage of follicular development at the time of PGF injection.

Lot of variation has been reported in onset of estrus following administration of PGF2α which is mainly attributed to the ovarian follicular status. Therefore, a PGF protocol does not facilitate fixed time insemination of cows. To facilitate fixed timed insemination, GnRH and Estradiol based protocols have been developed which are based on exogenous control of follicular wave emergence. Therefore, it's important to understand the role of ovarian follicular waves in estrus synchronization.

3.3 FOLLICULAR WAVES

- Follicles are blister-like structures that grow on the ovaries. Each follicle contains an unfertilized egg that will be released to the oviduct if the follicle ovulates. The follicular growth occurs in waves throughout the estrous cycle.

- Each wave is characterized by rapid growth of numerous small follicles. From this wave of follicles, one follicle is allowed to grow to a much larger size than the others (12 to 15 mm). This large follicle is called the dominant follicle because it has the ability to regulate and restrict the growth of other smaller follicles. A few days after reaching maximum size, the dominant follicle begins to regress. As the dominant follicle regresses, it looses the ability to restrict the growth of other follicles.

- Thus, a new follicular wave is initiated coinciding with the regression of the previous dominant follicle. From the new follicular wave, another dominant follicle will be selected. Most cows will have two or three follicular waves during an 18 to 24 day cycle.

3.3.1 Follicular Waves and PGF

- Any dominant follicle has the capacity to ovulate provided the inhibitory effects of progesterone can be removed at an opportune time. Prostaglandins serve this function by destroying the CL, however, PGF has no direct effect on the normal pattern of follicular waves. Thus, the stage of follicular development at the time of PGF injection will affect the interval from injection to standing estrus.

- Animals injected when the dominant follicle is in the growing phase will display estrus within 2 to 3 days, whereas animals with aged or regressing dominant follicles (C) may require 4 to 6 days before a new follicle can be recruited for ovulation.

3.3.2 Follicular Waves and GnRH

- An injection of GnRH causes a release of Luteinizing Hormone (LH) from the pituitary gland in the brain. This LH "surge" results in ovulation or luteinization of most large dominant follicles. A new "synchronized" follicular wave is initiated in these animals 2 to 3 days later. Because GnRH stimulates development of luteal tissue in place of the dominant follicle, a higher percentage of cows will possess sufficient luteal tissue to respond to PGF 7 days later. Injecting cows with PGF 7 days after a GnRH injection synchronizes luteal regression in animals with previously synchronized follicular development. The result is a higher estrus response rate and much better synchrony of estrus as compared to PGF alone.

- Although GnRH synchronizes follicular development in most cows, some cows do not respond to the first GnRH injection. If the GnRH injection fails to luteinize a follicle in animals that were due to show heat naturally around the time of the PGF injection, the treatment fails to prevent those animals from displaying estrus as they normally would. Research in both beef and dairy cows has consistently revealed that 5 to 10% of cows treated with GnRH will display standing estrus 6 to 7 days later. These natural heats should be bred when detected and subsequent injections are not administered. GnRH-based synchronization protocols are not currently recommended in virgin heifers because they do not respond to GnRH injections as consistently as do mature cows.

3.4 GnRH-PGF BASED SYNCHRONIZATION PROTOCOLS

- Numerous new synchronization protocols currently recommended for cows use gonadotropin-releasing hormone (GnRH) in conjunction with PGF. Each GnRH-based protocol uses the same basic framework, which involves an injection of GnRH followed 7 days later with an injection of PGF.

- The way animals are subsequently handled for heat detection and breeding is where the protocols begin to vary. It is important to understand the concept of follicular waves in cattle to understand the benefits of GnRH-based synchronization protocols and how they work.

3.4.1 Select Synch

- With the Select Synch System, cows are injected with GnRH and PGF 7 days apart. Heat detection begins 24-48 hours before the PGF injection and continues for the next 5-7 days. The PGF injection is excluded for cows detected in estrus on day 6 or 7. Animals are inseminated 8 to 12 hours after observed in standing estrus. Alternatively, heat detect and A.I. until 48 to 60 hours after PGF and then mass-AI the rest of the herd at 72 hours and give GnRH to those cows that have not exhibited estrus.

- Major benefits of the Select Synch system are simplicity and tighter synchrony of estrus. Most animals will display standing estrus 2 to 4 days after the PGF injection. Overall, estrus response rates in well-managed beef herds average ~70 to 75% with no adverse effect on conception rates (60 to 70%), resulting in synchronized pregnancy rates that average between 45 and 50%.

- Select Synch followed by heat detection and 72 hour fixed time A.I. allows producers to maximize potential pregnancy rates while minimizing labor requirements for estrus detection (7,8). Heat detection is used to catch the early cows and to breed the majority of the herd (60 to 70%) to standing heats. Estrous detection can be terminated at 48 to 60 hours after PGF followed by mass-AI of the non-responders at 72 hours with GnRH. This option gives all cows an opportunity to conceive and, compared to strict fixed-time AI options such as Ovsynch and Cosynch, drug costs are reduced as only 30 to 40% of the herd will receive the second GnRH injection. Additionally, if less than 40 to 50% of the herd is detected in estrus by 72 hours, the mass mating can be aborted, saving drugs, money and semen that might otherwise be wasted on anestrous cows.

- Select Synch resulted in more cows in standing estrus, equal or better conception rates and ultimately more cows pregnant during the synchronized breeding period. These benefits were particularly evident in the anestrous cows where estrous response rates were improved by 25% and conception rates (66%) were comparable to those of cycling cows. The Select Synch system more than doubled the percentage of anestrous cows that became pregnant during the synchronized breeding period.

3.4.2 Ovsynch

- Ovsynch is a fixed-time AI synchronization protocol that has been developed, tested and used extensively in dairy cattle . The protocol builds on the basic GnRH-PGF format by adding a second GnRH injection 48 hours after the PGF injection. This second GnRH injection induces ovulation of the dominant follicle recruited after the first GnRH injection. All cows are mass inseminated without estrous detection at 8 to 18 hours after the second GnRH injection. Across large numbers of dairy cattle, pregnancy rates to Ovsynch generally average in the 30 to 40% range. Although these numbers may not appear impressive at first, it is important to understand them in terms of an applied reproductive management program.

- Ovsynch pregnancy rates in dairy herds can be significantly improved if cows are set-up or "pre-synchronized" to be in the early luteal phase of the estrous cycle at the time of the first GnRH injection. This can be accomplished with 2 injections of PGF given at 14-day intervals with the last injection administered 12 to 14 days prior to starting Ovsynch.

- Although Ovsynch allows for acceptable pregnancy rates with no heat detection, it does not eliminate the need for heat detection. Ovsynch treated animals should be observed closely for returns to estrus 18 to 24 days later. Additionally, natural heats can occur on any given day and as many as 20% of cows will display standing estrus between days 6 and 9 of the Ovsynch protocol. Conception rates in these animals will be compromised if bred strictly on a timed AI basis.

3.4.5 Cosynch

Although Ovsynch has proven to be a reliable timed AI program for beef cows as well, Ovsynch requires four trips through the working chute. Research at Colorado State University demonstrated that comparable pregnancy rates can be achieved with only animal handlings by breeding all cow coinsiding with the second GnRH injection. Thus, the name Cosynch. As with any fixed time AI protocol, results to Cosynch can be variable, but in general range from 40 to 50%. As with Ovsynch, pregnancy rates are maximized if the early heats are visually detected and bred using the AM/PM rule.

3.5 MGA - PGF SYSTEM

The MGA-PGF system is a time tested, proven method for synchronizing estrus in beef and dairy heifers. Melengestrol Acetate (MGA) is a synthetic form of the naturally occurring hormone, progesterone. For best results, mix MGA with 3 to 5 lbs of a grain supplement and feed at a rate of 0.5 mg/ head/day for 14 days. Top dressing or mixing MGA in a TMR can work, but intake (and thus results) tends to be more variable. Within 3 to 5 days after MGA feeding, most heifers will display standing heat. DO NOT BREED at this heat as conception rates are reduced. Wait 17 to 19 days after the last day of MGA feeding, and inject all heifers with a single dose of PGF. For the next 5 to 7 days, inseminate animals 8 to 12 hours after detected estrus. Success of the MGA system depends on adequate bunk space and proper feeding rates so the appropriate dosage is consumed by each heifer on a daily basis.

With good heat detection of well-managed heifers at the proper age, weight and body condition, you can expect to achieve synchronized pregnancy rates of 50 to 70%.Because the synchrony of heats following the MGA-PGF protocol can be variable, pregnancy rates to single, fixed time inseminations are also variable. However, very acceptable pregnancy rates (45 to 55%) have been achieved to a single insemination at 72 hours or by double inseminating at 60 and 96 hours following the PGF injection.

- Heat detect & AI for 3 to 5 days after removal
- Fixed-time AI & GnRH at 50 to 60 hours after removal
- Heat detect & AI 72 hours and fixed-time AI of non-responders with GnRH at 72 to 80 hours after removal.

3.5.1 Eazi-Breedtm CIDR® Applications

⦿ The EAZI-BREED CIDR is a T-shaped vaginal insert that delivers the natural hormone progesterone during the 7-day treatment period. Cows and heifers receive Lutalyse (5 mL) on day 6 or 7after CIDR insertion with CIDR removal on day 7.

⦿ Females are bred 8 to 12 hours after observed estrus for the next 3 to 5 days or at a single fixed time 48 to 64 hours after CIDR removal. Research indicates the extra animal handling to give Lutalyse on day 6 versus day 7 may reduce the average interval to estrus by about 12 hours with a slight improvement in synchrony of response, but will have no impact on the overall estrous response rate.

⦿ Numerous research trials indicate an injection of GnRH a t CIDR insertion may further improve synchronized reproductive performance, especially among anestrous cows. In other words, pregnancy rates of the many popular GnRH-PGF protocols such Ovsynch, CO-Synch and Select Synch are improved by inserting the CIDR at GnRH injection and removing the CIDR at the Lutalyse injection on day 7.

⦿ Breeding cows and heifers to detected estrus for 72 hours after CIDR removal, followed by timed AI of non-responders with GnRH appears to minimize the herd to herd variation in pregnancy rates by breeding most cows to standing estrus with a minimum investment in estrus detection labor, while the timed AI gives all females the opportunity to conceive.

3.5.2 MGA - Select

⦿ The MGA-Select system superimposes the MGA heifer protocol on the Select Synch protocol. Cows are fed MGA (0.5 mg/ head/day) for 14 days and treated with Select Synch starting 12 days after the last day of MGA feeding. As with Select Synch, cows are bred to observed heats for 72 to 80 hours after PGF and non responders are mass-mated with a concurrent injection of GnRH (Option 1).

⦿ Alternatively, cows may be mass-mated with a concurrent GnRH injection at 72 to 80 hours after PGF. The MGA feeding helps to "jump start" cyclicity in many anestrous cows and presynchronizes cycling cows for optimum response to Select Synch. Numerous studies indicate the MGA Select system yields outstanding synchroinzed A.I. pregnancy rates ranging from 55 to 65% with both heat detection and fixed time A.I. breeding options.

⦿ As with the heifer protocol, do not breed cows detected in estrus within 10 days of MGA feeding. ®MGA is a registered trademark of Pfizer Animal Health and is not approved for use in lactating dairy cows.

3.6 MANAGEMENT TIPS TO MAXIMIZE SUCCESS

- The major factor affecting the success of any estrus synchronization protocol is the percentage of animals cycling at the initiation of treatment.

- The single most important factor affecting cyclicity is nutrition. Feed cows to achieve a moderate or better body condition score by the time of calving and increase energy levels in rations to minimize the body condition loss.

- Perform all vaccinations at least three weeks ahead of the synchronization and breeding period to provide ample time for the immune system to respond and provide protection from the disease in question.

- First-calf heifers, late calving cows, difficult births, and retained placentas are all associated with reduced fertility. Group these "high risk" animals separately so maximum nutrition and veterinary care can be efficiently provided.

4

ARTIFICIAL INSEMINATION: CURRENT AND FUTURE TRENDS

4.1 INTRODUCTION: AN OVERVIEW

- Artificial insemination (AI) is the manual placement of semen in the reproductive tract of the female by a method other than natural mating. It is one of a group of technologies commonly known as "assisted reproduction technologies" (ART), whereby offspring are generated by facilitating the meeting of gametes (spermatozoa and oocytes). ART may also involve the transfer of the products of conception to a female, for instance if fertilization has taken place in vitro or in another female. Other techniques encompassed by ART include the following: in vitro fertilization (IVF) where fertilization takes place outside the body; intracytoplasmic sperm injection (ICSI) where a single spermatozoon is caught and injected into an oocyte; embryo transfer (ET) where embryos that have been derived either in vivo or in vitro are transferred to a recipient female to establish a pregnancy; gamete intrafallopian transfer (GIFT) where spermatozoa are injected into the oviduct to be close to the site of fertilization in vivo; and cryopreservation, where spermatozoa or embryos, or occasionally oocytes, are cryopreserved in liquid nitrogen for use at a later stage.

- AI has been used in the majority of domestic species, including bees, and also in human beings. It is the most commonly used ART in livestock, revolutionising the animal breeding industry during the 20th century. In contrast to medical use, where intra-uterine insemination (IUI) is used only occasionally in human fertility treatment, AI is by far the most common method of breeding intensively kept domestic livestock, such as dairy cattle (approximately 80% in Europe and North America), pigs (more than 90% in Europe and North America) and turkeys (almost 100% in intensive production). AI is increasing in horses, beef cattle and sheep, and has been reported in other domestic species such as dogs, goats, deer and buffalo. It has also been used occasionally in conservation breeding of rare or endangered species, for example, primates, elephants and wild felids. The other ARTs in animals are generally confined to specialist applications or for research purposes, since the cost would be prohibitive for normal livestock breeding. In contrast, IUI is used less often in human fertility treatments than IVF or ICSI.

4.2 ADVANTAGES AND DISADVANTAGES OF ARTIFICIAL INSEMINATION

AI in animals was originally developed to control the spread of disease, by avoiding the transport of animals with potential pathogens to other animal units for mating and by avoiding physical contact between individuals. The use of semen extenders containing antibiotics also helped to prevent the transmission of bacterial diseases. The advantages and disadvantages of AI are as follows:

4.2.1 Advantages

- ⊙ AI helps prevents the spread of infectious or contagious diseases, that can be passed on when animals are in close contact or share the same environment;
- ⊙ The rate of genetic development and production gain can be increased, by using semen from males of high genetic merit for superior females;
- ⊙ It enables breeding between animals in different geographic locations, or at different times (even after the male's death);
- ⊙ Breeding can occur in the event of physical, physiological or behavioural abnormalities;
- ⊙ AI is a powerful tool when linked to other reproductive biotechnologies such as sperm cryopreservation, sperm sexing;
- ⊙ AI can be used in conservation of rare breeds or endangered species.

4.2.2 Disadvantages

- ⊙ Some males shed virus in semen without clinical signs of disease ("shedders").
- ⊙ Some bacterial pathogens are resistant to the antibiotics in semen extenders or can avoid their effects by forming bio-films;
- ⊙ There has been a decline in fertility in dairy cattle and horses associated with an increase in AI;
- ⊙ The focus on certain individuals may result in loss of genetic variation.

4.3 VIRUSES IN SEMEN

Cryopreserved semen doses can be "quarantined" until the male is shown to have been free of disease at the time of semen collection. In contrast, the short shelf-life of fresh semen doses means that they must be inseminated into the female before the disease-free status of the male has been established. Breeding sires used for semen collection are tested routinely for the presence of antibodies in serum as being indicative of past infection, but some viruses, e.g. equine arteritis virus, may be shed in semen for several weeks before there is evidence of sero-conversion. In other cases, usually of congenital infection, individuals may be permanent virus "shedders" without ever developing antibodies. Semen from these individuals represents a source of pathogens for disease transmission to naive females.

4.4 BACTERIA IN SEMEN

Normally, in a healthy male, the ejaculate itself does not contain microorganisms, but contamination occurs at semen collection from the prepuce and foreskin, the male´s abdomen and the environment. Semen processing from livestock usually takes place without access to a laminar air flow hood, resulting in potential contamination from the laboratory environment. Antibiotics are added to semen extenders to limit the growth of these contaminants and prevent disease in the inseminated female. Although the female reproductive tract has well-developed physiological mechanisms for dealing with contamination introduced during mating, these can be overwhelmed by bacteria multiplying in semen extenders or where semen is deposited in a non-physiological location.

AI revolutionized animal breeding in the 20th century, particularly in combination with sperm cryopreservation. The AI industry has developed dramatically in most domestic species in the last few decades and its use is now widespread in intensive animal production. The development of other associated technologies, such as sperm selection and sex selection, are predicted to create powerful tools for the future, both for domestic livestock breeding and for the purposes of conservation. AI will continue to play a role in fertility treatment for human patients, although it may be superseded by IVF or ICSI. It has been suggested that AI (in animals) is entering a new era where it will be used for the efficient application of current and new sperm technologies.

4.5 ANTIBIOTICS IN SEMEN EXTENDERS

The addition of antibiotics to semen extenders is controlled by government directives, both nationally and internationally, which state the types of antibiotic to be used and also their concentrations. In general, there is a tendency to use broad spectrum, highly potent antibiotics in various combinations to reduce sperm toxicity. However, these antibiotics may exacerbate the development of resistance, both for the people handling the semen extenders and in the environment during the disposal of unused extenders or semen doses. The scale of the problem becomes apparent if one considers that approximately four million liters of boar semen extender containing antibiotics are used in Europe alone per year.

4.6 PRE-REQUISITES FOR AI

Pre-requisites for AI include a supply of semen, reliable methods for oestrus detection in the female and a means of inserting the semen into the female reproductive tract.

4.6.1. Collection of Semen

- In most domestic animals, semen is collected by means of an artificial vagina, for example, bull, ram, stallion, after allowing the male to mount either an oestrous female or a phantom.

- The artificial vagina consists of a lubricated liner inserted into an outer jacket, the space between the two being filled with warm water. The pressure can be increased by adding air.

- The ejaculate is deposited into an insulated collecting vessel attached to one end of the liner.

- Boar and dog semen is usually collected by manual stimulation.

- In some species that are accustomed to being handled, it is possible to obtain semen by vaginal washing after natural mating, for example, dogs and marmoset monkeys. However, in this case the spermatozoa have already been exposed to vaginal secretions which may be detrimental to sperm survival.

- Human males can usually supply a sample by masturbation, except in the case of spinal injury when electroejaculation may be necessary. Some other primates can be trained to supply a semen sample on request in the same manner.

- For other species, for example, most non-domestic species, electroejaculation represents the only possibility for obtaining a semen sample.

- The problem with electroejaculation is that the secretions of the accessory glands may not be present in the usual proportions, which may have a detrimental effect on sperm survival.

4.6.2 Constituents of Semen

- Semen consists of spermatozoa contained in a watery fluid known as seminal plasma that represents the combined secretions of the different accessory glands, such as the seminal vesicles, bulbourethral gland and prostate. The relative contributions of these different glands vary between species. In some species, such a most primates, the semen coagulates immediately after ejaculation and then liquefies over a period of approximately 30 minutes.

- In most other species, the ejaculate remains liquid, the exception being in camelids where the seminal plasma is highly viscous and does not liquefy readily *in vitro*. The addition of enzymes has been suggested as a means of liquefying primate or camelid semen. However, all the enzymes tested thus far (collagenase, fibrinolysin, hyaluronidase and trypsin) have been seen to cause acrosomal damage in spermatozoa and are contra-indicated if the spermatozoa are to be used for AI. Recent advances have shown that camelid semen, extended 1:1 volume to volume, will liquefy in 60-90 min at 37 °C.

⊙ Seminal plasma contains an energy source (often fructose), proteins and various ions such as calcium, magnesium, zinc and bicarbonate. Seminal plasma not only activates the spermatozoa, which have been maintained in a quiescent state in the epididymis, but also functions as a transport medium to convey the spermatozoa into the female reproductive tract and to stimulate the latter to allow spermatozoa to swim to the site of fertilization. It has been suggested that seminal plasma, at least in horses, is also a modulator of sperm-induced inflammation, which is thought to play an important role in sperm elimination from the female reproductive tract.

⊙ Various proteins in the seminal plasma, such as spermadhesins and the so-called CRISP proteins (CRISP = cysteine-rich secretory proteins) are thought to be associated with sperm fertility. It is likely that these proteins bind to spermatozoa immediately, setting in motion a sequence of intracellular events via a second-messenger pathway. In some species, small membrane-bound vesicles have also been identified in seminal plasma, apparently originating from different accessory glands in various species. These vesicles, variously named prostasomes, vesiculosomes, or epididysomes depending on their origin, fuse with the sperm outer membrane, increasing motility and possibly being involved in sperm capacitation and acquisition of fertilizing ability. However, their exact mechanism of action has yet to be elucidated.

⊙ Seminal factors promote sperm survival in the female reproductive tract, modulate the female immune response tolerate the conceptus, and to condition the uterine environment for embryo development and the endometrium for implantation. The mechanism of action in the endometrium is via the recruitment and activation of macrophages and granulocytes, and also dendritic re-modelling, that improve endometrial receptivity to the implanting embryo. Cytokine release has embryotrophic properties and may also influence tissues outside the reproductive tract.

⊙ Exposure to semen induces cytokine activation into the uterine luminal fluid and epithelial glycocalyx lining the luminal space. These cytokines interact with the developing embryo as it traverses the oviduct and uterus prior to implantation. Several cytokines are thought to be involved, for example granulocyte-macrophage colony stimulating factor (GM-CSF), a principle cytokine in the post-mating inflammatory response, targets the pre-implantation embryo to promote blastocyst formation, increasing the number of viable blastomeres by inhibiting apoptosis and facilitating glucose uptake. Interleukin-6 (IL-6) and leukocyte inhibitory factor (LIF) are similarly induced after exposure to semen.

⊙ Clinical studies in humans showed acute and cumulative benefits of exposure to seminal fluid but also a partner-specific route of action. Live birth rates in couples undergoing fertility treatments are improved if women engage in intercourse close to embryo. The use of seminal plasma pessaries by women suffering from recurrent spontaneous abortion is reported to improve pregnancy success. Partner-specificity of the response is suggested by increased rates of preeclampsia in pregnancies from donor oocytes or semen when prior exposure to the donor sperm or conceptus antigens has not occurred.

4.6.3 Semen Processing

Although seminal plasma plays such an important role in activating spermatozoa and in the female reproductive tract, it is detrimental to long-term sperm survival outside the body. Under physiological conditions, spermatozoa are activated by seminal plasma at ejaculation and then swim away from the site of semen deposition in the female. It is only during *in vitro* storage that spermatozoa become exposed to seminal plasma long-term. Thus it is customary to add a semen extender to the semen, to dilute toxic elements in seminal plasma, to provide nutrients for the spermatozoa during *in vitro* storage and to buffer their metabolic by-products. The addition of extender also permits the semen to be divided into several semen doses, each containing a specific number of spermatozoa that has been determined to be optimal for good fertility in inseminated females.

4.6.4 Semen Preservation

Semen is used either immediately after collection ("fresh") for example turkeys, human beings; after storage at a reduced temperature ("stored") for example horses, pigs, dogs; or after freezing and thawing ("cryopreservation") for example, bulls.

4.6.5 Fresh Semen

In contrast to animal species, human semen is not extended prior to processing (see previous section) and is not usually kept for more than a few hours before use. Poultry semen cannot be extended as much as is customary for other species since the spermatozoa are adversely affected by increased dilution. Goat semen cannot be kept at 37 °C because an enzymatic component of the bulbo-urethral gland secretion hydrolyses milk triglycerides into free fatty acids, which adversely affects the motility and membrane integrity of buck spermatozoa. For liquid preservation, goat semen can be stored at 4 °C although fertility is retained for only 12-24h. The rate of extension used for stallion semen varies between countries but rates of 1:2, 1:3 or even 1:4 (v/v) semen:extender are common. The standard practice in some countries is to have 500 million or one billion progressively motile stallion spermatozoa for fresh or cooled semen doses respectively. Boar semen doses contain three billion progressively motile spermatozoa.

4.6.7 Stored Semen

Storing extended semen at reduced temperature helps to extend sperm life by slowing their metabolism as well as by inhibiting bacterial growth. Bacteria grow by utilizing the nutrients in semen extenders, thus competing with spermatozoa for these limited resources, and release metabolic byproducts, thus creating an environment that is not conducive to maintaining viable spermatozoa. Furthermore, as bacteria die, they may release endotoxins that are toxic to spermatozoa. However, cooled stored semen is the method of choice for breeding horses and pigs, enabling the semen dose to be transported to different locations for insemination. Stallion semen is stored at approximately 6 °C while boar semen is stored between 16 and 18 °C.

Most boar semen doses are sold as cooled doses. In contrast, some stallions produce spermatozoa that do not tolerate cooling, rapidly losing progressive motility. In such cases, the only option currently is to use fresh semen doses for AI immediately after semen collection, although a new method of processing, centrifugation through a single layer of colloid, has been shown to solve the problem.

4.6.8 Cryopreservation

Semen is most useful for AI if it can be cryopreserved, since this method of preservation ideally enables the semen to be stored for an unlimited period without loss of quality until needed for AI. Since the frozen semen does not deteriorate, it can be quarantined until the male has been shown to be free from disease at the time of semen collection. However, the spermatozoa of various species differ in their ability to withstand cryopreservation: ruminant spermatozoa survive well whereas poultry spermatozoa do not, with less than 2% retaining their fertilizing ability on thawing. For farm animal breeding, the cost of cryopreservation and the likelihood of a successful outcome following AI must be considered when deciding whether to use fresh, cooled or frozen sperm doses.

The spermatozoa are mixed with a protective solution containing lipoproteins, sugars and a cryoprotectant such as glycerol. These constituents help to preserve membrane integrity during the processes of cooling and re-warming. However, sperm motility must also be maintained, so that the thawed spermatozoa can reach the oocytes after insemination and fertilize them. In most species, the seminal plasma is removed by centrifugation before mixing with the cryoextender, for example, stallion, boar, goat and human semen. The extended semen is packed in straws and frozen in liquid nitrogen vapour before plunging into liquid nitrogen for long-term storage. There is considerable variation in the success of sperm cryopreservation between different species, despite intensive research into the constituents of cryoextenders and the rates of cooling and re-warming. Human spermatozoa can be frozen relatively successfully using commercially available cryoextenders and programmable freezing machines.

4.7 OESTRUS DETECTION AND OVULATION

Successful AI also depends on depositing the semen in the female tract at around the time of ovulation. Like human beings, some domestic animals breed throughout the year, for example cattle and pigs, but others show a defined period of reproductive activity known as the breeding season, for example sheep and horses. The onset of the breeding season is controlled by photoperiod. Both of these patterns of reproductive behaviour are characterised by waves of ovarian activity, culminating in ovulation. However, in some other species ovulation occurs in response to the stimulus of mating, for example, cats, rabbits and camels. In spontaneously ovulating species, ovulation occurs at some time during, or shortly after, oestrus, which is the period of time when the female is receptive to the male. Since a successful outcome for AI depends on the deposition of spermatozoa at a suitable time relative to ovulation, oestrus detection is crucial if the female is to be inseminated at the correct time. Males of the same species are, of course, very good at detecting oestrus females, but since many livestock breeding units that practice AI do not have male animals in the vicinity, it is essential that husbandry personnel become good at recognising oestrous behaviour.

Although some domestic animals may show well-developed oestrous behaviour, e.g. dairy cows, others may not. Behavioural signs of oestrus in cows include restlessness or increased activity, vocalization, chin resting, swelling of the vulva, vaginal discharge and mounting other cows, although there are breed differences in the frequency and intensity of these signs. In sheep and goats, vulval swelling and vaginal discharge may be seen, and there is usually pronounced male-seeking behaviour. When AI is to be used in sheep, it is usual to synchronize oestrus with hormones: intravaginal sponges impregnated with progestagens are inserted to suppress the ewe´s natural ovarian cycle for 12 days. On sponge removal, pregnant mare serum gonadotrophin is administered, with AI taking place at a set time thereafter. Alternatively, a vasectomised ram wearing a marker can be run with the females. When the females are in oestrus, the vasectomised ram marks them as he mounts, thus enabling them to be identified for AI. Oestrous sows and mares can be identified by the behaviour exhibited towards teaser males.

4.7.1 Induced Ovulation

When AI is performed in species that are normally induced ovulators, such as rabbits, cats and camels, it is necessary to stimulate ovulation. The easiest way to achieve this stimulation is to mate the female with a vasectomised male, but this practice is not desirable from the point of view of disease control and necessitates having vasectomized males available. The most acceptable alternative is to administer luteinising hormone, usually in the form of human chorionic gonadotrophin. However, the major disadvantage is that repeated injections of this foreign protein may cause the female to develop antibodies, thus inactivating subsequent doses.

4.7.2 Artificially Induced Ovulation

Hormones may be administered to spontaneous ovulators to ensure that ovulation occurs at the correct time relative to AI. However, since 2006, the use of hormones in food-producing animals has been forbidden in the European Union, and local regulations may also apply in other parts of the world. Previously most dairy goats in France were inseminated out of the breeding season with deep frozen semen, after induction of oestrus and ovulation by hormonal treatments. This protocol provided a kidding rate of approximately 65%. As an alternative to administering artificial hormones, out-of season breeding may be induced by altering the photoperiod or by introducing a buck to the herd. This practice is also widespread in intensive sheep flocks.

4.7.3 Deposition of Semen in the Female

There are differences between species in the site of semen deposition during natural mating. In ruminants and primates, semen is deposited in the vagina whereas in pigs, dogs, camels and horses, semen deposition is intrauterine. In most species, it is possible to pass an insemination catheter through the cervix, thus enabling semen to be deposited in the uterus during AI. Exceptions are sheep and goats, where the tightly folded nature of the cervix does not permit easy passage of an insemination catheter. The advantages of depositing the semen in the uterus are that the spermatozoa have less far to travel to reach the oviducts and fewer spermatozoa are lost through back-flow. A smaller volume of semen can be used per insemination dose than for intravaginal deposition, thus permitting an ejaculate to be divided into several AI doses, and the cervix, which can act as a barrier to the passage of spermatozoa, is bypassed. A disadvantage, particularly for human IUI, is that seminal plasma is also introduced into the uterus, unless specific steps are taken to separate the spermatozoa from seminal plasma before IUI.

4.8 SPECIES DIFFERENCES IN THE USE OF AI

Despite the fact that the basic principles of AI are the same in all species, there is wide variation in the uptake of this biotechnology in different species.

4.8.1 AI in Cattle

In cattle, frozen semen doses are used most widely in Europe and North America, since there are well-established protocols for cryopreserving bull semen. Semen doses typically contain approximately 15 million motile spermatozoa. In New Zealand, however, fresh semen doses are used instead, with AI occurring within 24h of semen collection.

4.8.2 AI in Pigs

The porcine AI industry uses liquid semen that has been stored for one to several days at 16-18°C. In contrast, AI with cryopreserved boar spermatozoa results in lower farrowing rates and litter sizes than with cooled, stored spermatozoa, making the use of frozen-thawed sperm doses unattractive for commercial pig breeders. Exceptions to this rule are when semen is transported over long distances, which creates problems in temperature regulation, and in instances where it is vital that the boars can be shown to be free of disease at the time of semen collection. The ability of boar spermatozoa to survive cool storage so well is attributed to low levels of reactive oxygen species (ROS) in semen or to the efficient scavenging of ROS by anti-oxidative components in seminal plasma.

4.8.3 AI in Horses

AI has increased in horses in the last 25 years. Initially, fresh semen was used for AI shortly after semen collection, but nowadays the use of cooled semen has largely replaced fresh semen in Europe and North America. The extended semen is cooled to approximately 5 , and transported in insulated containers, together with a cold pack. The fertility of the cooled semen is maintained for approximately 24h. Frozen semen doses are used infrequently, although this trend may change with the development of better freezing protocols. However, with the increased use of cooled semen, a concomitant decrease in foaling rate has been observed in several countries, such as Finland and Sweden, although the reason for this apparent decline in fertility is unknown. Unlike bulls and boars, which are selected for their semen quality as well as for their potential "genetic merit" in production characteristics (body composition, weight gain, milk production etc), the choice of stallions as breeding sires is based solely on their performance in competition. Thus, considerable variation in semen quality exists between stallions. This variation, coupled with increased use of a wider range of stallions, may be contributing to the observed decline in foaling rate. Other important considerations are the lack of established standard methods for cooling and freezing of stallion spermatozoa, for the sperm concentration in the insemination dose, or for quality control of raw or frozen/thawed spermatozoa.

4.8.4 AI in Sheep

Ram semen differs from stallion and boar semen in consisting of a small volume (a few mL) of seminal plasma containing a very high concentration of spermatozoa. In Europe, reproductive research in livestock has tended to focus on cattle and pigs rather than on small ruminants, with the result that sperm handling and cryopreservation for AI is less advanced in the latter species. In addition, the anatomy of the female reproductive tract in these species presents more of a barrier to successful insemination than in cattle, since the cervix is tightly folded, making insertion of the insemination catheter difficult. Productivity in sheep and goats could be increased, by improving the quality of the spermatozoa assigned for use in AI, and improving the AI techniques in these species. Recent innovations in sheep breeding include the development of a flexible catheter at the National Center for Genetic Resource Preservation, Fort Collins, Colorado, that can be inserted through the ovine cervix, thus overcoming the barrier to effective AI in this species.

AI in sheep and goats is traditionally performed with fresh or cooled spermatozoa, with acceptable fertility results. However, use of foreign breeds, genetic improvement and the use of "safe" semen from other countries requires the use of frozen semen, to enable analyses for contaminants or diseases in the "donor" male to be completed before the semen doses are used for AI. Although the post-thaw motility of frozen semen from goats and sheep is usually considered acceptable, low fertility has been associated with its use in AI, mainly owing to a shortened lifespan of the spermatozoa.

4.9 INTRAUTERINE INSEMINATION IN HUMAN FERTILITY TREATMENT

It is estimated that 10-20% of couples wanting to conceive are unable to do so without some assistance. In 40% of cases, sub-fertility is due to female factors, with a further 40% being due to male factors. The remaining cases may be multifactorial or idiopathic in origin. The use of IUI is generally contraindicated in male factor infertility, with IVF or ICSI being the treatments of choice. Since spermatozoa must be able to reach the site of fertilization and the products of conception must be able to reach the uterus for implantation, female factor infertility due to blockage of the oviducts is better treated by IVF or ICSI than by IUI. The patient's own semen or donor semen may be utilized for these fertility treatments.

4.10 AI - STATE OF THE ART

AI can help to improve reproductive efficiency in animals for food production or sport. We are living in a world of scarce resources where there is constant competition for water, food, land and energy. Since protein of animal origin continues to be one of the most important forms of nourishment for human beings, animals are an essential part of the ecosystem and must be husbanded in a sustainable fashion. Animal production not only "competes" with human beings for the aforementioned resources, but also produces large amounts of effluent and gaseous emissions which can affect the environment. Therefore, it is vital for the survival of the planet that all aspects of animal production are justified and optimized. Through grazing or browsing and the recycling of nutrients, animals also contribute to maintaining the landscape in a productive state.

The production of food of animal origin is based on breeding offspring to enter various husbandry systems. Therefore, one of the first points for optimization is in increasing reproductive efficiency, using an holistic approach. Females should be bred for the first time at an appropriate age to ensure the birth of healthy offspring and optimum lactation, without compromising the health of the female. Subsequent breeding attempts should also be timed appropriately to balance the metabolic requirements of lactation and early pregnancy. Females not conceiving or showing early embryonic loss should be identified at an early stage for re-breeding or culling. However, optimizing female reproduction demands a supply of spermatozoa. The spermatozoa must be readily available (i.e. can be stored), robust, and capable of fertilization, initiation of early embryonic development and regulation of placental formation, and there must be a means of delivery to an appropriate site in the female.

4.11 AI IN OTHER SPECIES

AI in non-domestic species presents several new challenges compared with domestic species. In many cases little is known about the reproductive biology of the species in question, and handling the animals may cause them stress, with the attendant risk of injury. The animals must be managed correctly for the establishment and maintenance of pregnancy. There are reports of successful AI in deer, buffalo and camelids.

4.12 FUTURE TRENDS IN AI

It is highly probable that the use of AI in livestock will continue to increase. AI not only facilitates more effective and efficient livestock production, but can also be coupled to other developing biotechnologies, such as cryopreservation, selection of robust spermatozoa by single layer centrifugation, and sperm sex selection.

4.12.1 AI in Increasing the Efficiency of Livestock Production

Apart from some specialist sheep or goat units focussing on milk production for cheese and intensive meat production, farming of these species tends to be confined to marginal land that is unsuitable for crop production or grazing for dairy cattle. There has been limited selection for production traits. However, there is a resurgence of interest in them now in developed countries because of growing awareness that small ruminants could represent better utilization of scare resources than larger ones, such as cattle, while producing less methane and effluent. In many developing countries, sheep and goats are better suited to the climate than cattle, and it is culturally acceptable to eat their meat and milk products. Thus it is likely that there will be an upsurge in the use of AI in sheep and goats in the future, with an emphasis on improving production traits by the introduction of superior genes. However, it is essential that any A.I. scheme aimed at large scale improvement of the national herd must be supported by improved animal husbandry and animal health, otherwise the pregnancies resulting from AI will not go to term, and the offspring will either not survive or will fail to thrive. Many of the advanced ART are of little help in areas where basic husbandry skills are inadequate.

4.12.2 Biomimetic Sperm Selection

One potential disadvantage of AI is that the natural selection mechanisms within the female reproductive tract to select the best spermatozoa for fertilization may be bypassed when AI is utilized. Biomimetics is the use of technologies and/or processes that mimic a naturally occurring event. Several *in vitro* procedures have been suggested that could be used to mimic selection of good quality spermatozoa in the female reproductive tract and thus fit the definition of biomimetics in ART. These include sperm processing procedures such as swim-up, sperm migration, filtration and colloid centrifugation. Of these methods, the one that is most applicable to livestock and human spermatozoa is colloid centrifugation.

4.12.3 Density Gradient Centrifugation

Human spermatozoa for fertility treatment are usually processed to remove the seminal plasma and to select those of better quality. In most cases, this is achieved either by sperm migration, in which the more motile spermatozoa are separated from the rest of the ejaculate, or by density gradient centrifugation, where the most robust spermatozoa are selected. The benefits of density gradient centrifugation are as follows:

- ◉ Poorly motile and abnormal spermatozoa are removed,
- ◉ Sources of ROS (cell debris, leukocytes, epithelial cells and dead or dying spermatozoa) are removed;
- ◉ Sperm survival is improved during frozen and non-frozen storage;
- ◉ Bacterial contamination is controlled without antibiotics.

4.12.4 Single Layer Centrifugation

Density gradient centrifugation is seldom used when processing animal semen because of the limited volume of semen that can be processed at one time and the time taken to prepare the different layers. A novel sperm preparation technique, Single Layer Centrifugation (SLC) through a colloid, was developed at the Swedish University of Agricultural Sciences (SLU) to select the most robust spermatozoa from ejaculates. This method is similar to density gradient centrifugation (DGC), but is better suited for animal semen since it has been scaled-up to process whole ejaculates.

4.13 SEX SELECTION

For many centuries, animal breeders and researchers have endeavoured to control the sex of the offspring born, for various reasons. Initially male offspring were preferred for meat production, because of the better feed conversion efficiency and lean-to-fat ratio of males, whereas females were preferred for dairy purposes, except that some males of high genetic merit were still required as sires. Couples may want a child of a specific sex to avoid the expression of sex-linked disorders.

Many methods have been proposed for separating X- and Y-chromosome bearing spermatozoa, based on physical properties, e.g. size of the sperm head, or functional properties e.g. swimming speed. However, the only method which has been shown to work reliably is that of selection and separation of spermatozoa whose DNA is stained with a bis-benzimidazole dye, H33342, using the sorting capacity of a flow cytometer (Morrell et al., 1988; Johnson et al., 1989). This method functions because the X chromosome is larger than the Y, therefore taking up more of the DNA-specific stain and showing a higher fluorescence when the spermatozoa are passed through a laser beam. In bulls, for example, the difference in DNA content between the X and Y- chromosome is approximately 4.2%. However, the process of sorting sufficient numbers for an insemination dose in the flow cytometer takes too long, since the stained spermatozoa must pass one at a time through a laser beam for detection of their DNA content. Moreover, the pregnancy rate after insemination of sexed bull spermatozoa is lower than with unsexed spermatozoa, making the procedure inefficient and expensive. Experience has shown that the staining profiles are highly individual, with the result that it is not possible to separate the X- and Y-chromosome bearing spermatozoa efficiently from all males.

Alternative methods of sex selection are also being investigated. A company in Wales, Ovasort, has identified sex-specific proteins on the sperm surface and have raised antibodies to them. It is intended to use the antibodies to aggregate spermatozoa bearing a specific sex chromosome, thus enabling them to be removed from the general population.

A combination of ARTs would also be relevant for sperm sexing. Thus, the speed of flow sorting can be increased by first removing the dead and dying spermatozoa from the population, for example by density gradient centrifugation or single layer centrifugation. Such a combination may increase the "sortability" of sperm samples. Sufficient sexed spermatozoa may be obtained from flow sorting for IVF, thus generating embryos or blastocysts for subsequent transfer. However, methods of speeding up the selection process are needed if flow cytometry is to become useful for species other than the bovine.

4.14 SPERM CRYOPRESERVATION

As previously mentioned, the ability of cryopreserved spermatozoa to retain their fertilizing ability varies widely between species. New cryoextenders and new protocols are being developed constantly in an effort to address this issue. One recent advance has been the introduction of dimethylsulphoxide and the amides formamide and dimethylformamide as cryoprotectants, in place of glycerol. These molecules seem to function better than glycerol for some individuals whose spermatozoa do not freeze well, for example, some stallions. One explanation for this observation is that these molecules are smaller than glycerol and therefore may cause less damage when they penetrate the sperm membrane. However, no method appears to be universally successful within one species. As far as turkey spermatozoa are concerned, it seems that the development of a successful freezing method will require more than new cryoprotectants and additives.

4.15 REMOVAL OF VIRUSES FROM EJACULATES

Viral infectivity can be removed from the semen of patients with viral infections such as HIV and hepatitis, by a sequential method of sperm preparation i.e. centrifugation on a density gradient followed by a "swim-up". Spermatozoa from virally infected men prepared by this method have been used in assisted reproduction attempts, apparently without sero-conversion of mothers or children. However, some studies with HIV report that density gradient centrifugation alone will not remove all viral infectivity. Since spermatozoa may function as vectors for viruses, further work is required to investigate how closely different viral particles are associated with the sperm membrane with putative carry-over during processing. The double method of processing has also been successful in removing equine arteritis virus from an infected stallion ejaculate in a preliminary study. SLC together with swim-up was used to reduce viral infectivity from boar semen spiked with porcine circo virus .

4.16 AI IN CONSERVATION BIOLOGY

It has been suggested that AI and other forms of ART could be useful for genetic conservation and preservation of rare breeds. Many of these technologies have been successful to some degree in a research setting, but none have produced results sufficient to effect population-wide improvements in genetic management. Cryopreservation of semen has been the most widely applied ART in this respect, but much of the frozen semen in so-called gene banks has never been tested for fertility. A lack of suitable females or dearth of knowledge about the reproductive biology of the species involved may contribute to this deficit. However, long-term storage of frozen gametes of unknown fertility is not a sustainable policy for the conservation of rare breeds and endangered species. The development of *in vitro* methods of testing sperm fertility would contribute considerably to conservation efforts. Since the semen quality in these animals may be poor, techniques such as SLC of samples prior to AI could be of considerable benefit in conservation breeding.

5

SEMEN QUALITY AND FERTILITY AFTER ARTIFICIAL INSEMINATION

5.1 INTRODUCTION

Artificial insemination (AI) is an assisted reproductive technology that is very important in intensive breeding and production of cattle and swine. AI is commonly used on a global basis; in Finland some 90% of cows and 80% of sows are artificially inseminated. In cattle, the AI is usually performed using cryopreserved semen as bull spermatozoa maintain their viability very well during the freezing-thawing process. On the other hand, the success rate for fertilization of sows with frozen-thawed semen is poor, so swine AI is usually performed with doses stored in a liquid state at +15-20 °C for max 3-5 days. To achieve acceptable results with AI, one needs to be successful in every procedural step from semen collection, dilution and storage to inseminating at the optimal time regarding estrus and ovulation.

Assessment of in vivo fertilizing capacity of semen represents a challenge because it is influenced not only by semen-related factors but also by female fertility and by many other factors that may or may not be determinable (Amann and Hammerstedt 2002). Due to the complexity of the fertilization process, several sperm attributes are required for successful fertilization, such as the ability to undergo capacitation, hyperactivation, the acrosome reaction, binding to the zona pellucida, and oocyte penetration. Despite the limitations as predictors of fertility, evaluation of sperm morphology and progressive motility is the most common method used to assess viability of fresh and frozen-thawed semen at AI stations.

The importance of using low sperm numbers for AI to initially determine relative fertility in vivo has been confirmed in a number of studies. This approach is likely to avoid the potential compensatory effect when using high sperm numbers per AI dose. This compensation can, however, be only partial, and some sperm defects are clearly uncompensable. In practice, the possibility of using reduced sperm numbers for insemination in the field is limited due to potentially lowered fertility, which can cause marked economic losses to farmers. Another limiting factor in clinical trials is the wellbeing of the animals. It is especially relevant when studying factors harmful for the animal itself, as is the case with mycotoxins. Despite the limitations of large-scale field trials, they remain the only way to study the efficacy of different treatments under commercial conditions that laboratory assessment cannot adequately duplicate.

Farm animals in Finland are dependent on stored feed and bedding during the 7 to 8 month indoor feeding season. The microbiological quality of hay varies according to weather conditions during harvest and storage. In humid conditions, both bacteria and fungi may colonize hay and produce various toxins. These microbial impurities in feed and bedding enter farm animals orally and through inhalation.

The fungal genera most frequently reported to produce mycotoxins with adverse effects on animal health are Fusarium (T-2 and HT-2 toxins, zearalenone), Aspergillus (aflatoxins, ochratoxin), Stachybotrys (satratoxin), and Penicillium (ochratoxin). Clinical mycotoxicosis is rare in Finland, but low doses of mycotoxins in feed and bedding can cause subclinical symptoms, such as decreased fertility. The occurrence of microfungi on Finnish dairy farms and found Fusarium spp. to be common in grain and straw. However, neither the occurrence of mycotoxins in Finnish hay nor their subclinical manifestations in farm animals are well studied.

Many contagious animal diseases cause reproductive problems worldwide, but Finland has been almost free of many of these, including Bovine Respiratory Syncytial Virus (BRSV). In winter 2000, however, a major outbreak of BRSV occurred, spreading to the quarantine section of a rearing station for young dairy bulls intended for use in AI. BRSV is a pneumovirus and an important component of the calf pneumonia complex. The most severe disease is observed in calves less than 6 months old, but it is also occasionally isolated from adult cattle with acute respiratory disease. BRSV is widely distributed in most countries. A BRSV outbreak was recently associated also with fibrotic lesions in bull testes.

The pig is considered to be, at least partly, an intrauterine ejaculator. Therefore, deposition of the semen in the uterus may enhance reproductive success compared with using the caudal portion of the cervix as the primary site of semen deposition. Usually intrauterine insemination has been practiced in order to allow for a reduction in the number of sperm per dose. There is little information available to indicate whether intrauterine insemination with a standard AI dose is beneficial.

High quality semen is crucial for successful AI. Quality is, however, influenced by many factors that may or may not be determinable. This thesis concentrates on semen quality and on some factors affecting it in dairy bulls and boars, with emphasis on field fertility. The investigations were based on laboratory assessments and large field trials, as well as on historical datasets from Finnish AI companies and the breeding organization (FABA). This study resulted in the five original papers presented at the end of this thesis.

5.2 ARTIFICIAL INSEMINATION

High reproductive performance is a key factor for optimal economic success in cattle and swine production. AI is the oldest and currently most common assisted reproductive technology and an important tool in animal production. Originally AI was introduced as a means of preventing spread of venereal diseases. Today AI represents a much more cost-effective means of disseminating superior genes. AI has been most widely used for breeding dairy cattle; 253 million frozen AI doses and 11.7 million liquid doses are produced worldwide every year. In Finland, all bull semen used for AI is cryopreserved, allowing long storage times and easy distribution, and inseminations are generally done by trained inseminators.

The quality of semen used for AI is crucial to its outcome. Assessment of in vivo fertilizing capacity of semen presents a challenge because it is influenced by many different sources a variation, which may or may not be determinable. Despite the limitations of large-scale field trials, they are still the only way to study the efficacy of various treatments under commercial conditions that laboratory assessment cannot accurately substitute for. It focuses on different aspects affecting male reproduction. We developed a new method for sperm viability determination, studied the deleterious effects of trichothecenes in feed and BRSV infection on sperm quality as well as studied the importance of semen quality and insemination dose for reproductive success.

The extent of AI use in the pig industry varies greatly among countries. AI accounts for 80% of litters in Finland. Over 19 million inseminations of gilts/sows are performed worldwide each year, almost all of them (99%) with liquid semen stored at +15-20 °C for up to 3-5 days (cooled semen), but this figure is expected to rise.

The AI industry has to deal with a time lag between semen collection and insemination and subsequent fertilization. Storage of semen doses for a certain time is necessary for their distribution and to optimize efficient use of semen for AI. It is of practical and economic importance that the semen storage time does not negatively influence fertility. However, the natural ageing process cannot be prevented in liquid diluted boar semen, not even during the first days of storage. Spermatozoa progressively lose viability when stored in a semen extender at ambient temperature. A suppression of spermatozoal metabolic activity, to reduce energy consumption and by-product formation, is needed to ensure sperm longevity. Maintaining extended semen at a temperature between 15 °C and 20 °C has been reported as optimal for storage of liquid boar semen. This practice is widely used and was followed also in the boar experiments in this study.

As a generalization, some 40-50% of the sperm population in mammals does not survive cryopreservation even with optimized protocols. When comparisons are made on the basis of similar numbers of motile (assumed viable) spermatozoa, results are still generally poorer than with fresh semen, indicating that even the viable subpopulation after cryopreservation is compromised. Boar spermatozoa are very sensitive to cold shock, possibly because of the low cholesterol/phospholipid ratio of their membranes. Therefore, the success of fertilization with frozen-thawed semen differs significantly between bull and boar. Another important observation related to cryopreserved boar semen is the timing of ovulation in the pig, which can occur over an extended period of estrus such that spermatozoa may be required to survive up to 40 h in the oviduct. Waberski et al. (1994a) noted that fertility with cryopreserved semen can be high providing that the insemination is carried out within 4 h before ovulation. Outside this period, fertility with cryopreserved spermatozoa declined substantially, but fresh semen maintained its fertility for a much longer period. Cryopreserved spermatozoa do not survive as long as fresh spermatozoa in the female genital tract. These factors explain the use of liquid (fresh) semen in pigs and cryopreserved semen in cattle.

5.3 SEMEN EVALUATION

When choosing a male for breeding, especially for AI, it is imperative to assess its potential fertility by undertaking clinical and laboratory examinations. The *in vitro* semen evaluation, complementary to the clinical examination, is of high diagnostic value for assessing testicular and epididymal function, and/or the genital tract of the male, allowing elimination of clear-cut cases of infertility, or potential sub-fertility. Likewise, the degree of normality of the semen before being processed for AI can be analyzed. The semen analysis routinely includes an immediate assessment of volume, appearance (i.e. color, contamination, etc.), sperm concentration and motility, as well as later determination of sperm morphology and the presence of foreign cells. Once screened for normality, ejaculates preserved for AI are assessed for sperm concentration and sperm motility. These are the parameters most often used to determine sperm viability in post-thaw semen samples as well as to estimate breeding potential of a sire under field conditions. Unfortunately, neither a simple semen analysis nor the routine evaluation post-thaw enable the determination *a priori* of the potential fertility level that the analyzed semen will reach, particularly after AI. The usefulness of these parameters to measure fertility of a semen sample accurately is controversial and correlations between sperm motility and fertility have revealed large ranges of variation. Correlations between sperm morphology and fertility have also been found vary widely, and have most often been statistically non-significant when the semen of AI quality grade has been assessed. Researchers have also used additional laboratory assays to predict accurately the fertilizing potential of a semen sample. Individual laboratory assays, which evaluate a single parameter, are not effective predictors of fertility. However, a combination of several assays may provide a better prediction of fertility. The testing of a large number of parameters should lead to a higher accuracy because fertilization is a multi-factorial process. However, most of these analyses are expensive and time-consuming and cannot be applied under field and/ or commercial conditions. In conclusion, sperm analysis conducted under commercial conditions leads to the detection of ejaculates of very poor quality. However, the pre-selection of the samples, the high number of sperm per dose and the high quality of the semen used in the AI programs reduces the variability, giving a low probability of detecting fertility differences associated with seminal parameters.

5.3.1 Sperm Concentration

Accurate and precise determination of sperm concentration in an ejaculate is important for AI stations in order to produce uniform insemination doses containing an adequate number of sperm. A certain safety margin is often used by AI stations to ensure that all insemination doses contain a minimal number of sperm. This also implies that some insemination doses contain an excessive number of sperm and that males of high genetic value are not used efficiently. This safety margin also affects the average revenue per ejaculate for the AI station.

The hemocytometer has often been referred to as the "gold standard" for assessing sperm numbers. The equipment is slow, however, and multiple measurements of each sample are needed to obtain a precise result. The use of a spectrophotometer is probably the most frequent method used by AI stations for assessment of sperm concentration. For satisfactory results, periodic calibration of hemocytometers is necessary. The detection spectrum is limited for these instruments, and accurate quantification of sperm numbers in dilute or concentrated samples is problematic. Spectrophotometers overestimate sperm numbers in dilute semen samples and underestimate sperm numbers in concentrated sperm samples. For individual raw ejaculates of boar semen, differences in the amount of gel particles or debris (cytoplasmic droplets, bacteria) can result in an inaccurate determination of the sperm concentration. Electronic particle counters allow rapid determination of sperm concentration but tend to include any debris in the size range of sperm. Fluorometric measurements of the amount of DNA, using DNA-specific fluorochromes have been investigated, but this method requires stoichiometric staining.

5.3.2 Motility

Most frequently, the semen quality of dairy bulls and boars in AI centers is evaluated using sperm concentration and motility in fresh semen and motility in post-thaw samples for bulls. While some authors established a correlation between motility and field fertility.

Good progressive motility of spermatozoa is an indicator of both unimpaired metabolism and intactness of membranes. Estimation of motility has fundamental importance in daily quality control of semen. The percentage of motile spermatozoa is used to calculate the required degree of dilution and to estimate the number of intact spermatozoa per insemination dose. Regular motility checks of boar semen after dilution and during the holding period furnish information on the capacity for preservation of the semen of each boar and its individual peculiarities. Motility is mostly assessed of all DNA and minimal unspecific fluorescence from the extender.

Visually with a light microscope. It is inexpensive and quick, but accuracy depends on the subjective estimation by individuals even though surprisingly consistent results can be obtained. Objective Computer Assisted Sperm Analysis (CASA) systems have become commercially available, but these systems are not frequently used in commercial AI-centers because of the high investment costs. Encouragingly small sampling errors and high correlations with fertility have been reported, but the reported procedures have to be applied to an independent dataset to test their repeatability. The main problem in CASA systems is related to the standardization and optimization of the equipment and procedures. A simple visual estimation of sperm motility remains a useful tool for routine semen assessment for research purposes and in the AI industry.

As boar spermatozoa show a higher percentage of circular movement than those from other species, except stallions, it is recommended to estimate the different forms of motility, including proportions of progressive spermatozoa. Estimates undertaken using phase contrast microscopy within 20-30 min of dilution cannot be integrated easily into the production processes. Stored boar semen should be examined regularly and motility values above 60% should be considered satisfactory.

5.3.3 Morphology

Morphological abnormalities of sperm can have a detrimental impact upon fertilization and embryonic development. Bulls and boars used for commercial AI are selected to a certain degree on the basis of a low incidence of morphologically abnormal spermatozoa, so that statistical calculations concerning their correlation with fertility are not very informative, although some evidence for a relationship between sperm morphology and fertility in bulls has been presented. A complete morphological examination is recommended when bulls and boars are introduced into the AI station and during subsequent regular routine examinations. Principles for determining sample size for morphological assessment of spermatozoa were extensively discussed. The percentage of cytoplasmic droplets in boar ejaculates used for AI should not exceed 15%, especially when stored semen is used. In addition to the incidence of cytoplasmic droplets, the percentage of other morphological alterations should not exceed 20%.

A number of classification systems exist for morphological abnormalities of sperm, including i) primary and secondary defects, which classify sperm abnormalities on the basis of their presumptive origin; ii) major and minor defects, a revised system where sperm defects are classified in terms of their perceived adverse effects upon male fertility; and iii) compensable and uncompensable semen traits according to a theoretical increase in numbers of functionally competent sperm that will or will not solve the problem. A compensable defect is one where the defective spermatozoa either do not reach the site of fertilization, or fails to initiate the fertilization process. Defects that lead to failed fertilization or early pregnancy loss are termed uncompensable.

5.3.4 Fluorescent Methods / Assessment of the Plasma Membrane Status

Plasma membrane status of spermatozoa is of outmost importance due to its role, not only as a cell boundary, but also for cell-to-cell interactions, e.g. between spermatozoa and the epithelium of the female genital tract and between the spermatozoon and the oocyte and its vestments. The relationship between the degree of sperm damage post-thaw and fertility is not always clear, but tends to increase when damage is extensive or when fertility values are widely spread. Fluorescent viability staining in semen evaluation serves many purposes depending on the used combination of fluorochromes, such as determination of the sperm membrane integrity, acrosomal status, or function of mitochondria. Fluorophore-incubated spermatozoa have been mostly studied with fluorescence microscopy (where an operator is required for counting). It is a simple and cheap method, but one that only allows assessment of a few hundred spermatozoa per sample. Sperm counting can be markedly increased using a fluorescence-activated cell-sorting instrument (FACS) where thousands of spermatozoa can be examined in minutes, reaching correlations with *in vitro* and *in vivo* fertility. However, the costs of purchase and running this equipment are quite high. Alternatively, computerized fluorometry can be used to evaluate membrane integrity of large sperm numbers yielding significant, albeit variable, correlations with fertility.

The usual approach in fluorescent viability staining is to use two fluorophore stains that react with the same cellular constituent – one stain that identifies only living sperm and another that stains only dead (or moribund) sperm, like membrane-permeant (SYBR-14) and impermeant stains (PI) together. Using a fluorometer, either rapid freezing and slow thawing or detergents are required to induce membrane damage as detected by PI in all sperm cells to create a totally killed subsample. Measuring simultaneously the fluorescence of the sample and the fluorescence of the totally killed subsample allows calculation of relative values.

Based on plasma membrane studies, the viability of post-thaw ejaculates varies within and between bulls, and a correlation between sperm viability after thawing and fertility has been demonstrated, although the predictive value is limited. In pigs, plasma membrane integrity parameters in liquid semen stored for seven days correlated significantly with motility and fertility parameters (non-return rate and litter size) in multiparous sows, but not in gilts with synchronized estrus.

5.4 THE NUMBER OF SPERMATOZOA / INSEMINATION DOSE

The number of sperm in the insemination dose is an important factor affecting the probability that a female will become pregnant after AI, and in litter-bearing animals also the litter size. To maximize pregnancy rate, the number of sperm in a dose is intentionally set high, but this management approach tends to obscure differences among males (or treatments) that might impact outcome of breeding when fewer sperm are used. Certain males achieve maximum fertility after AI with very few motile sperm (e.g. 1 million for cattle), whereas for other males 20-30x more motile sperm are required to maximize fertility. At high sperm numbers per AI dose individual bulls differ in their maximal NR%. That is unrelated to the rate at which they approach this maximum. *Vice versa*, subfertile bulls could not be restored to normal fertility by increasing numbers of sperm per inseminate. Data for cattle are most comprehensive, but it would be erroneous to assume that this principle, which results from so called "compensable defects" of sperm, is not operational in other species. Actually, it has been stated by several authors that insemination trials with reduced sperm numbers are needed to reveal subfertile males and/or to detect differences between males.

From the perspective of validating a diagnostic assay, the use of an excessive number of sperm when measuring fertility increases the probability that the compensable defects in sperm will be masked. A compensable defect is one in which low fertility can be overcome, at least in part, by increasing the number of sperm in the AI dose. Low fertility caused by an uncompensable defect persists regardless of the number of sperm per insemination. Hence, with a compensable defect of sperm, the "problem" causing low fertility results from the failure of sperm characteristics being expressed before sperm enter the oocyte. An uncompensable defect involves an attribute (or attributes) being expressed only after a spermatozoon enters an ovum. When a spermatozoon with an uncompensable defect fertilizes an oocyte, it is unable to complete the fertilization process or sustain embryonal development, so pregnancy may not be detected.

There is an increasing interest among AI/breeding organizations to decrease the number of spermatozoa per straw to be used for AI, related to economic revenues and the expected increased use of sex-sorted semen in bulls. It is generally accepted that a total of 15×10^6 spermatozoa in a frozen 0.25 ml straw is enough to achieve an acceptable fertilization rate in cattle provided that post-thaw motility is equal to or above 50%. Extension of semen to low sperm numbers per AI-dose has been related to a decrease in bull sperm viability *in vitro* with significant bull variation.

In AI of swine several dose regimens are applied, ranging from 1.5×10^9 to 6.0×10^9 spermatozoa per intra-cervical insemination dose. A lower sperm dose is more profitable for AI centers and makes more effective use of superior boars. However, when decreasing the insemination dose, the effect of semen quality becomes more important and otherwise compensable morphological deficiencies can no longer be overcome. This leads to decreased fertility rates and smaller litter sizes.

5.5 INTRAUTERINE (TRANSCERVICAL) INSEMINATION IN SOWS

The pig is considered to be, at least partly, an intrauterine ejaculator. Deposition of the semen in the uterus may enhance reproductive success compared with the standardized insemination procedure termed intra-cervical insemination that involves deposition of the semen dose in the posterior portion of the cervical canal by means of a catheter that engages with the posterior folds of the cervix, simulating the corkscrew tie of the boar's penis. The standard insemination is a simple, inexpensive and quick procedure, but requires a large number of spermatozoa per dose (generally more than 2.5×10^9 cells), of which approximately 30-40% flow back within 1 h of insemination. The intrauterine insemination technique was developed to overcome this event and improve the number of spermatozoa able to reach the uterotubal junction and sperm reservoir in the isthmus.

To perform intrauterine (transcervical) AI, a thin and semi-rigid insemination device is passed through a conventional catheter previously inserted between the cervical folds. As the specialized inner insemination device is 15-20 cm longer than a conventional catheter, it can extend over the remaining folds of the cervix and enter the uterine body (Watson and Behan 2002; Roca et al. 2006). Criticism for probable traumatic injury indicated by the presence of blood in the vulva after insemination, which has been reported in some animals, could be caused by incorrect manipulation of the device. The device should always be inserted carefully and not forced if some resistance is encountered. One important limitation is that the method is unsuitable for insemination of gilts because of difficulties in passing the device through the cervix.

Intrauterine insemination has been usually practiced in order to allow for a reduction of the number of sperm per dose, which is especially important with sex-sorted or frozen-thawed spermatozoa. A similar technique has been developed to allow transcervical embryo transfer. In field trials comparing this technique using cooled semen and reduced sperm numbers (1×10^9 spermatozoa / dose) or conventional AI (3×10^9 spermatozoa / dose), farrowing rates have been similar. However, it has been accompanied with a reduction in the number of piglets born per litter. When an even greater reduction of sperm dose has been attempted (0.5×10^9 sperm / dose), both farrowing rate and litter size have been poor.

The two major reasons why the sperm numbers can be somewhat lowered using intrauterine insemination without a reduction in farrowing rates are the full passage of the semi-rigid insemination device past the cervical folds and a substantial reduction in semen backflow to less than 20% of inseminated spermatozoa. However, the reduction in the number of piglets born per litter indicates that 1×10^9 is not an adequate number of spermatozoa to achieve high fertility with intrauterine insemination under farm conditions, and a higher number of spermatozoa / dose is suggested.

5.6 ASSESSMENT OF REPRODUCTIVE PERFORMANCE / FIELD FERTILITY

The most appropriate assessment of reproductive performance will vary depending on whether emphasis is placed on semen quality, differences among females or comparison of different AI strategies. In semen quality studies, reproductive success is often evaluated using the likelihood of conception after a particular AI. Of the alternative outcomes after copulation or AI, non-pregnant or pregnant, pregnant is a better estimate of the normalcy of sperm function and non-pregnant of abnormal sperm function. In this thesis we used a 60-day non-return rate to estrus (NR%) as the outcome variable for AI with bull semen, and farrowing rate and litter size for boar semen. It can be questioned whether NR% is an appropriate measurement for monitoring fertility, but the assessment of pregnancy rate, which would be more precise, requires that all animals in the herd are pregnancy tested, which is not practical or economical in large field studies where the farms are located throughout the country. For the calving rate, there is a 9 month delay for data which is impractical for study purposes. For all types of assessments of reproductive performance, there are some potential systematic errors, including culling and selling of animals that one needs to be aware of when drawing conclusions.

5.7 SEASONALITY

5.7.1 Cattle

Reproductive strategy in a seasonal breeder results in births during the spring when climate and food supplies are favorable for early postnatal development. Although cattle are not seasonal breeders in the strict sense of distinct seasons of reproductive activity and inactivity, there is evidence for seasonality in bovine reproduction. Several studies demonstrated the effect of season on fertility in cattle, and long-term statistics from Finland show a similar trend for higher fertility of cows during summer months with long but not too warm days, compared with winter, similarly as in Sweden. Extended photoperiods were also shown to hasten the onset of puberty in prepubertal heifers, as well as milk yield in dairy cattle.

5.7.2 Swine

Swine have been shown to be seasonal breeders with reduced NR% and litter size as well as increased early pregnancy loss during late summer - early autumn in a temperate climate like Finland. It is reported photoperiodic influences on sperm quality and libido in boars. It has been noted that a short-day length stimulates the pubertal maturation of spermatogenesis, while a long-day reduces the sensory scores for boar taint at slaughter in whole male pigs, demonstrating the broad effects of changing light patterns mediated by changes in melatonin secretion.

5.8 MYCOTOXINS / TRICHOTHECENES

Many types of mold are able to form toxic secondary metabolites termed mycotoxins. *Fusarium* molds are probably the most important mycotoxin producers that infect cereals in northern temperate regions. *Fusarium* molds are known to produce different mycotoxins, including trichothecenes such as deoxynivalenol (DON), 3-acetyldeoxynivalenol (3-AcDON), nivalenol (NIV), T-2 toxin (T-2), HT-2 toxin (HT-2), and also other toxins such as zearalenone (ZEN) in grains (Eskola et al. 2001). Some molds are able to produce more than one mycotoxin and some mycotoxins are produced by more than one mold species, and thus several mycotoxins are often simultaneously found in a single commodity. Despite the fact that in natural contaminations of grain and grain products with mycotoxins, different combinations of mycotoxin mixtures are often detected, research has largely focused on the toxic effects of single trichothecenes.

Cereals are the main source of trichothecenes and ZEN for consumers in the Nordic countries (Eskola et al. 2001). In Finnish cereals trichothecenes are more often found than ochratoxin A (OA) or ZEN. Mycotoxin contaminations in foods and animal feeds are usually heterogeneous, which causes difficulties in sampling. The method of sampling is very important: a sufficient number of equal sample portions should be taken at random points throughout the lot. Gas chromatography (GC) with electron-capture (ECD) or mass spectrometric (MS) detection is the most frequently used technique for trichothecene analysis today.

Exposure to mycotoxins has been associated with health problems in both humans and animals. The trichothecene mycotoxins are known to be potent inhibitors of protein synthesis, specifically in eukaryotes. The target organelle of trichothecenes is the 60S subunit of mammalian ribosomes. In mammalian cells, the trichothecenes inhibit DNA and RNA synthesis injuring organs with rapidly dividing cell populations such as germinal epithelium in testes. Furthermore, T-2 is a potent inducer of apoptosis. Symptoms and toxic effects on animals vary according to species, amount of toxin, and route of administration. The acute and chronic toxicities of trichothecenes are characterized by the depletion of lymphoid tissues. This feature indicates that they impair the immune system and modify immune responses. In cattle, T-2 toxin induces immunosuppression by decreasing serum concentrations of IgM, IgG, and IgA, neutrophil functions and lymphocyte blastogenesis, and the response of lymphocytes to phytohemagglutinin. This toxin was also shown to induce necrosis of lymphoid tissues. Other significant effects of trichothecenes are dermal toxicity, feed refusal, vomiting, diarrhea, intestinal hemorrhage, neurological disorders, heart lesions, alimentary toxic aleukia, hepatic or kidney damage, impairment of the hematopoietic system and alteration of the levels of biogenic amines such as dopamine and norepinephrine in the central nervous system. Bovine infertility and abortion in the final trimester of gestation have resulted from consumption of feed contaminated with T-2 toxin. In interstitial cells from testes of adult gerbils incubated with T-2, testosterone synthesis and secretion were dose-dependently inhibited. Similarly, degeneration and necrosis of spermatogenic cells in the semiferous tubules of guinea pigs have been described. Another characteristic of trichothecene toxicity is the high susceptibility of animals, when exposed by the inhalation route.

Generally, ruminants are less susceptible to trichothecene mycotoxicosis than monogastric animals. Rumen microorganisms, mostly protozoa, have been shown to deacetylate T-2 toxin to HT-2 toxin, which is less cytotoxic. The detoxifying capacity of the rumen microflora is saturable and varies with changes in the diet, or as a consequence of metabolic diseases, such as rumen acidosis. The metabolism of ingested material by the ruminal microbes may be considered as a first line of defense against toxic materials present in the diet. On the other hand, ruminants may be at a disadvantage if substances become toxic as a result of the action of ruminal microbes.

5.9 BOVINE RESPIRATORY SYNCYTIAL VIRUS (BRSV)

Bovine Respiratory Syncytial Virus (BRSV) is a pneumovirus belonging to the family Paramyxoviridae, subfamily Pneumovirinae, like its close relative Human Respiratory Syncytial Virus (HRSV). BRSV infection is an important part of the calf pneumonia complex causing up to 100% morbidity and 5-20% mortality in calves less than 6 months of age. The virus is occasionally isolated from adult cattle with acute respiratory disease, and can infect sheep. BRSV is widely distributed in most countries. Respiratory disease caused by BRSV is mainly observed in autumn-winter in temperate climates and is often diagnosed in combination with other viruses, bacteria or mycoplasmas.

The lability of BRSV in the environment has been underlined, but cell culture stocks of this virus have been reported to remain infective at 5 °C for 300 days. Investigations are lacking on the time of quarantine required to avoid transmission to sensitive animals. The infection dose might be much smaller than the amount of virus that is required for isolation *in vitro*. The mode of transmission during the cause of natural infection has not been defined, but direct contact is probably required.

It is not known exactly how long antibodies against BRSV remain in sera in adult cattle, but months or even years can pass without re-infection. In calves, maternal antibodies to BRSV have been documented to remain up to a maximum of 7 months of age. On farms where there are respiratory disease problems, including in Finland, BRSV seropositivity is frequently recorded. The overall incidence of BRSV in Finnish herds is unknown, but the outbreak in winter 2000 and minor outbreaks in the following winters suggest that the virus is currently widespread.

Incubation time for BRSV infection is estimated to be 2-8 days. Symptoms include cough, nasal discharge, and fever. Major BRSV induced lesions occur in the airways and lungs of calves, but viral RNA has also been demonstrated by reverse transcription-polymerase chain reaction (RT-PCR) outside the respiratory tract in lymphatic tissues and kidneys. RNA of BRSV has been found up to 71 days after an experimental infection of calves and in naturally infected cows in peripheral leucocytes and nasal mucosa by nested RT-PCR (nRT-PCR) in acute phase and again 4 weeks later. HRSV has been reported to be present in peripheral blood circulating mononuclear leucocytes of infected patients. Both HRSV and BRSV can spread in their hosts also outside the respiratory tract, but the viremic phase of infection is not routinely detected.

BRSV is present and replicates mainly in bronchial and alveolar epithelial cells on the luminal side of the respiratory tract. The virus infects several ciliated and non-ciliated epithelial cell types leading to an alteration of the ciliogenesis and partial or total loss of cilia. BRSV can replicate in a wide range of primary bovine cell cultures derived from the testis, turbinate, trachea, aorta, spleen and lung, as well as bovine and ovine alveolar macrophages, lymphocytes and peripheral monocytes and ovine testicular cells. After *in vitro* exposure to BRSV, the viability of lamb testis cells, but not of lymphocytes or monocytes, was significantly reduced as early as 24 h post exposure. In the same study, the lamb testis cells were the most permissive cells, with viral antigens present on 96 ± 2.2% of cells by 24 h post exposure and on all cells by 48 h post exposure.

BRSV infection in young (6-12 month old) bulls seems to increase testicular fibrosis by some unknown mechanism. It might have some immunological background similar to the lung pathology caused by RS viruses where fibrosis is common. Suggested that during the active process leading to fibrosis of testicular tissue spermatogenesis is adversely affected and this is later seen as poor sperm morphology.

5.10 AIMS

The quality of semen used in AI is crucial to the outcome. This is concentrates on semen quality and on factors affecting it, with emphasis on field fertility. It is based on laboratory assessments and large field trials as well as on historical datasets from Finnish AI companies and the breeding organization (FABA).

The specific aims were to:

- ⊙ Develop a new, easy-to-use and cost-effective method for sperm viability testing (i)
- ⊙ Investigate potentially harmful factors for semen quality and subsequent fertility in cattle (ii and iii)
- ⊙ Study the effect of sperm morphology in boars (iv)
- ⊙ Compare different ai doses in swine (iv)
- ⊙ Study the effect of two insemination methods on pig reproduction (V)

5.11 OVERVIEW MATERIALS AND METHODS

An overview of materials and methods is presented in this section. More detailed descriptions are available in the original publications (I-V). Clinical trials were carried out in commercial environments with standardized housing and management practices.

5.11.1 Animals and Management

Young bulls arrived in quarantine at 5 to 6 months of age, from farms where they had been born, and remained in quarantine for at least 30 days. Bulls were moved from quarantine to the rearing station at about 7 months of age and to one of two AI stations for semen collection for progeny inseminations at the age of 1 year.

The bulls (I-III) were of Finnish Ayrshire and Holstein-Friesian breeds and located at two bull stations. They were all between 12 and 36 months of age. The bulls were housed indoors and fed according to Finnish standards (in Finnish: MTT).

The boars were of Finnish Landrace and Yorkshire breeds (IV), and Duroc X Hampshire crossbred as well as pure Duroc and Hampshire (V). They were located at two boar stations. The age of the boars ranged from 9 to 40 months. The boars were housed indoors and fed according to Finnish standards (in Finnish: MTT).

The cows (I-III) were in commercial farms belonging to the national health control system. The sows in study IV were in commercial farms belonging to the health control system and in study V in a sow pool consisting of 440 sows housed in five herds, one of which was the nucleus herd for breeding and pregnancy. Three weeks prior to term, each group of 40 sows was transported to one of the four satellite herds for parturition and lactation. The satellite herds were located 30-80 km from the nucleus herd. The sow pool was a SPF system.

5.11.2 Semen Collection

Bull semen (I-III) was collected using the standard method, via an artificial vagina (2 ejaculates per bull per collection day). Semen from young bulls (13 to 18 months of age) was collected once a week, and from older bulls (over 18 months) twice a week, resulting in two or four ejaculates per week.

Boar semen (IV, V) was collected using a gloved hand technique no more than twice per week and the entire ejaculate was collected.

5.11.3 Semen Quality Assessment

Only grossly normal looking ejaculates were accepted for further evaluation and processing. The volume and density of the ejaculates were measured using a photometer (Novaspec II, Pharmacia LKB Biotechnology, Uppsala, Sweden) immediately after collection. Initial subjective progressive motility was estimated in all experiments and after freezing-thawing (I-III) by experienced technicians at the AI station. Motility was assessed with a phase-contrast microscope equipped with a heated stage, at 200x magnification. A drop of 10 μl of diluted semen was placed on a preheated (37 °C) glass slide and covered with a cover slip (22 x 22 mm).

The bull ejaculates were accepted for use in AI on the basis of their initial sperm concentration > 500 x 106 / ml, visual subjective sperm motility ≥ 60% and visual subjective post-thaw motility ≥ 40%. A batch consisted of two ejaculates (if both were acceptable, otherwise only one ejaculate) collected within a 15 minute interval.

Fresh boar ejaculates with total volume > 1 dl, progressive motility ≥ 60%, total number of spermatozoa ≥ 20 x 109 and total morphological abnormalities less than 20% of the sample were accepted. The average number of spermatozoa / AI dose was regularly controlled also in a hemocytometer (Bürker counting chamber, Fortuna, Germany).

5.11.3.1 Morphology

Morphology of semen samples was evaluated in studies II-IV. The smears were air-dried and sent to Saari laboratory, where they were fixed and stained using the Giemsa method according to Watson (1975); 100 spermatozoa / smear were examined, and classification of sperm morphology was performed as described by Blom (1983). Spermatozoa were divided into four classes: major sperm defects (e.g. pyriform head), proximal droplets, minor sperm defects (e.g. bent tail) and normal spermatozoa. Only the most serious sperm defect of each spermatozoon, based on its effect on fertility, was recorded. If there were less than 70% normal spermatozoa in the smear, an additional 300 spermatozoa were examined.

5.11.3.2 Sperm Membrane Integrity

Plasma membrane integrity of bull spermatozoa was studied (I) with fluorophore stain propidium iodide (PI) (Molecular Probes, Eugene, OR), which stains only dead or moribund cells. Simultaneous measurement of the fluorescence of the sample to be analyzed and the fluorescence of the totally killed subsample (rapidly frozen and slowly thawed) allowed calculation of relative values and the percentage of viable spermatozoa in the sample.

Two frozen semen straws from the same batch were pooled and dispensed into two vials after thawing. One of the vials from each batch was rapidly refrozen and slowly thawed to cause 100% disruption of the plasma membranes. The rapidly refrozen subsamples were then analyzed in the same manner and in the same black well plate as the non-treated samples.

Equal aliquots of Beltsville Thawing Solution (BTS) diluted sample and PI solution were dispensed into the well plate (Black Cliniplate, ThermoLabsystems, Helsinki, Finland) in three replicates. Blanks containing diluted extender (1:1 BTS and Triladyl) and PI were dispensed into the microtiter plate in four replicates. The plate was shaken gently for 2 min and incubated in the fluorometer for 8 min before analysis. Eleven samples and their blanks were then analyzed simultaneously.

Fluorescence was measured using an automatic computerized fluorometer (Fluoroscan Ascent, Labsystems, Helsinki, Finland). Both excitation and detection of fluorescence were carried out from the top of the well (reflectance fluorescence). The interference filter in the excitation path and that of the emission filter had their maximum transmission at 544 nm and 590 nm, respectively. The analysis was done twice for each batch.

Percentage of fluorescence was calculated from the ratio of fluorescence intensities in the sample and in the rapidly refrozen subsample, in relation to background fluorescence (blank) (Garner et al. 1997b), the blank being a combination of diluent and PI without spermatozoa.

Viability of the frozen-thawed batch was calculated as follows:

(1 - [fluorescence of the sample - blank] / [fluorescence of the rapidly frozen subsample - blank]) x 100%.

The maximal fluorescence output value of the rapidly refrozen subsample was calibrated against the total sperm count of the AI doses by the use of a hemocytometer in advance (Juonala et al. 1999). Thereby, the fluorometric measurements simultaneously provided total sperm count in the straws and viability of the spermatozoa.

For comparison of the fluorometer with fluorescence microscopy, samples were prepared and stained as described. In addition to analyses of the microtiter well plate with the fluorometer, the samples underwent microscopic evaluation with a fluorescence microscope (Olympus BH$_2$ with epifluorescence optics, Olympus Optical Co. Ltd., Tokyo, Japan) equipped with phase-contrast optics. Using only a little light, it was easy to visualize viable, unstained spermatozoa simultaneously with the fluorescent ones. From each sample 200 spermatozoa were evaluated. Only spermatozoa with completely unstained heads were considered viable.

5.12 INSEMINATIONS

In field trials, the cows (I-III) were inseminated in natural heat according to standard practice by trained inseminators. Similarly, the sows were inseminated in naturally occurring standing heat (IV-V). The sows were inseminated by farm owners (IV) or by technicians employed on the farm (IV-V). All experiments lasted at least a year to avoid bias caused by seasonal variation in fertility.

Frozen bull semen (I-III) was distributed throughout the country regardless of the AI station at which it was produced, and semen was used for inseminations only within the breed. The number of spermatozoa per straw was about 18 x 10^6.

In study IV, the age and breed-matched boars were randomly divided into two groups, with inseminations of 2 x 109 and 3 x 109 spermatozoa / dose, respectively. A sow was inseminated an average of 1.5 times / estrus.

In study V, the sows were transported to the nucleus herd on the day of weaning and housed in groups of 40 sows. After arrival at the nucleus herd, sows were checked for estrus symptoms twice a day. When in standing heat, sows were randomly allocated into either a uterine insemination group or a standard AI group and bred accordingly. In both treatment groups insemination was repeated once using semen from the same boar batch if the sow was still receptive 24 hours later. The sows were excluded from the study if not in estrus by day 6. The same technician performed both inseminations and the two technicians rotated intrauterine and traditional AI. In intrauterine AI, semen was deposited in the body of the uterus, whereas the caudal part of the cervix was used as the deposition site in the traditional AI. The catheters used were Verona (Minitüb, Tiefenbach, Germany) for the intrauterine AI and Goldenpig (IMV Technologies, L'Aigle Cedex, France) for the traditional AI. In both treatments 3×10^9 spermatozoa were included in each heterospermic dose.

5.13 FERTILITY PARAMETERS

Fertility was determined in clinical trials as the 60 day non-return rate (NR%) in dairy cows (I-III), and as the farrowing rate and litter size (total number of the piglets born / litter) in gilts and sows (IV-V). Fertility data in all experiments were obtained from the Agricultural Data-Processing Centre Ltd., Vantaa, Finland.

As in Norway, a year in Finland can be divided into four seasons based on the fertility of the cows: a good season in summer to autumn (June to October), two intermediate seasons, one in spring (April to May) and another in late autumn (November to December), and a poor one in winter (January to March) (personal communication, Finnish Animal Breeding Association FABA). In sows seasonal infertility occurs in Finland during late summer-early autumn (August-October). These seasonal variations in fertility are taken into account in statistical models in the experiments.

5.14 MYCOTOXIN INVESTIGATIONS

Feeding of the macroscopically suspicious hay to bulls (II) began on July 7. On October 17, the moldy hay was discarded and feeding with new hay of better quality was started.

The surface of the contaminated hay was sampled onto Scotch Tape® and inspected with bright field light microscopy at x 1000 magnification. A composite sample of hay from many hay bales was dissolved in acetonitrile and screened for the presence of T-2 toxin or zearalenone with a monoclonal antibody-based enzyme-linked immunosorbent assay (ELISA) (Toxiklon, Agricultural Biotechnology Center, Gödöllö, Hungary) as described by Barna-Vetro et al. (1994). Testing was done for T-2 and zearalenone in 3 and 2 replicates, respectively. The measurement ranges of the tests were 100 to 2000 ng / g for T-2 and 25 to 400 ng / g for zearalenone. The T-2 ELISA test cross-reacts with HT-2 toxin.

One sample of hay was also analyzed for *Fusarium* mycotoxins at the Finnish Food Safety Authority (Evira, Helsinki, Finland) using gas chromatography-mass spectrometry (GC-MS). The detection limit for all toxins tested was 20 ng / g.

5.15 BRSV STUDIES

At the beginning of 2000, a severe BRSV epizootic occurred in Finland, with even adult dairy cattle dying of pneumonia. In February 2000, the first outbreak of upper respiratory disease manifested as high fever, cough and nasal discharge in the quarantine area of the bull rearing station (III). Seven subsequent bull groups in quarantine were included in the study; four of these became infected, while the remaining three groups showed no signs of respiratory disease.

All young bulls from the above-mentioned seven subsequent quarantine groups that had passed the standard breeding soundness evaluation [i.e. physical examination, libido and semen quality (volume, motility, morphology)] at the AI stations were included in the study. When the animals were at the age of 14 ± 1 months, blood samples were taken for BRSV antibody testing. In addition, 68 older bulls already at the AI stations were randomly selected and sampled for BRSV antibodies. None of the old bulls showed any signs of respiratory disease. All antibody testing was done at the Finnish Food Safety Authority (Evira), Department of Virology (Helsinki, Finland), using a SVANOVIR RSV ELISA (SVANOVA Biotech AB, Uppsala, Sweden) method. Eleven bulls (12.2%) did not pass the breeding soundness evaluation, mainly because of poor semen quality (motility, morphology). One of these eleven bulls was azoospermic and had moderate adherences between the testis and *tunica vaginalis*.

5.16 STATISTICAL ANALYSES

The bull station, the season, and the breed served in statistical analyses (I) to explain variation in the number of sperm and in the percentage of viable sperm, as well as in the number of viable sperm in insemination doses. These factors, as well as the insemination number and parity, served to explain variation in NR%. When significant residual correlation existed between sperm parameters and non-return rates, those sperm parameters were included in the model as regressions to reveal their effect on NR%. For statistical analyses, the Least-Squares (LS) procedure was used (Harvey 1960) and means were expressed as LS means and standard error of means.

Statistical analyses (II) were carried out with the Statistix statistical software package, version 1.0 (Analytical Software, Tallahassee, FL). The Mann–Whitney U-test was used to compare morphology between young bulls in October 1998 and young bulls from previous years, and the Wilcoxon signed rank test for morphology in young bulls during different months.

The serological status for BRSV, bull station, insemination number (first vs. later ins station by BRSV status and season by BRSV status interactions served as variables in statistical analyses (III) to explain variation in NR%. The LS procedure was used, and results were expressed as LS means and standard error of means. The T-test was applied to compare morphology between BRSV seropositive and negative young bulls at the age of 14 months.

Table 1. Summary of trials.

Study	Inseminations (N)	Species	Breed	Parameter (S) Of Interest	Statistical Model	Aim
i	92120	Cattle	Ay, Fr	Viability, Nr%	Ls	Novel Assay
ii	-	Cattle	Ay	Motility, Morphlogy	U-Test, Signed Rank Text	Trichothecenes
iii	128 299	Cattle	Ay	Morphology, Nr%	Ls, T-Test	Brsv
iv	45 562	Swine	L, Y	Nr%, Litter	Logistic & Linear	Ai Does And Sperm
v	326	Swine	Hybrids (L; Y)	Farrowing Rate, Litter Size	Logistic & Linear Regression	Transcervical Ai
Ay=Ayrshire, Fr=Holstein-Friesian						
L=Landrace, Y=Yorkshire						
LS=Least-Squares						

Multiple regression models were used (IV) to assess the effect of the dose on fertility parameters. In the case of non-return rate, a logistic regression model was built, including dose, breed and semen characteristics as explanatory variables and the non-return rate as the outcome variable (R = 0.65). To study the effect of AI dose on fertility parameters, two separate linear regression models were used for first parity sows and older sows. In both cases, the model included dose, breed and semen characteristics as the explanatory variables and the non-return rate as the outcome variable (R = 0.45 for the first parity model and R = 0.41 for older parities). No interactions for the variables were noted. Furthermore, the analyses indicated no collinearity problem between the variables. For the analyses, SPSS (SPSS Inc., Chicago, USA) version 11.0 was used.

Sample size (V) was calculated based on the following assumptions. Expected difference in the means of the groups was set at 0.8 piglets (11.8 vs. 11.0 live born piglets / litter was assumed for the two treatment groups). Level of confidence was set at 95%, power of the study at 0.8 and expected standard deviation at 2.9 piglets / litter. Using these assumptions, an independent sample size of 165 sows per group was required in order to detect a significant difference between the treatment groups.

Using farrowing rate (farrowed or not) and live-born litter size (normal distribution checked for and found, repeat breeders included) as the outcome variables, a logistic and linear regression approach, respectively, was chosen to study the effect of the following factors: treatment, AI operator, breed, satellite herd preceding weaning, parity, weaning-to-estrus interval and length of lactation. For an effect to be included in the model, a conservative 0.2 level of significance was applied. All analyses were carried out using SPSS 13.0 for Windows (Lead Technologies, inc., U.S.).

5.17 FLUOROMETRIC STUDIES (I)

The fluorometric analyses were done in three replicates and twice for each batch. The method was precise and accurate when compared to fluorescence microscopy. In a comparison test the percentages (±SEM) of viable bull spermatozoa detected by the fluorometer (67.5 ± 1.48) and by the microscope (67.8 ± 1.34) were almost identical.

The raw means of the sperm numbers and the overall NR% are given in Table 2.

Table 2. Summary statistics for semen and fertility parameters of 436 bull semen batches.

	Mean ± SD	Min	Max
Sperm viability(%)	64.8 ± 7.9	33.8	81.7
Total number of sperm/does(x109)	18.2 ± 2.9	10.1	26.2
Total number of sperm/does(x109)	11.8 ± 2.2	5.71	19.0
NR%	71.1 ± 10.5	27.3	97.3

(70.0 ± 0.47) and highest in summer (75.3 ± 0.54) (P < 0.001).

A significant residual correlation existed between NR% and number of viable sperm in an insemination dose (R = 0.051, P = 0.016). The correlation between NR% and viability of spermatozoa (R = 0.046, P = 0.027) was also significant, albeit not significant between NR% and total number of spermatozoa per dose (R = 0.03, P = 0.147).

5.18 EFFECT OF TRICHOTHECENES IN THE HAY (II)

Many species of fungi had contaminated the hay, *Fusarium* spp. being some of the most frequent. In the immunoassay, T-2 toxin was detected in concentrations of 220, 300, and 600 ng / g. This was confirmed with monoclonal ELISA tests. One composite sample of hay, when analyzed using gas chromatography–mass spectrometry (GC-MS), showed elevated levels of T-2 toxin (47 ng / g) and very high amounts of HT-2 toxin (570 ng / g). No zearalenone toxin was detected with any of the methods used.

An increase of one million viable spermatozoa in an insemination dose increased NR% by 0.2%, P = 0.016. An increase of 1% in the rate of viable spermatozoa increased NR% by 0.05%, P = 0.027.

Feeding of the moldy hay lasted from July 7 to October 17. The decrease in sperm quality, as detected by low progressive motility and poor morphology persisted several months after withdrawal of the moldy hay. The percentage of rejected ejaculates was significantly increased over that of the previous year (Figure 1).

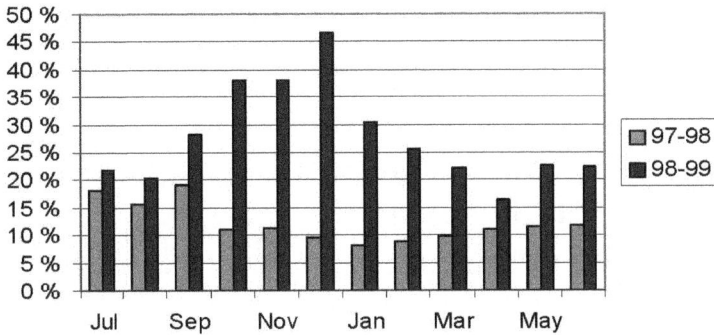

Figure 1. The average percentage of rejected bull ejaculates from July 1997 to June 1999.

Analyses of sperm morphology revealed that the ejaculates from October to December 1998 were inferior to those in breed- and age-matched bulls at the same AI station during previous years (Table 3). All forms of abnormal spermatozoa increased in number.

The number of spermatozoa per straw was about 18 x 106. Total number of spermatozoa in the accepted ejaculates remained unaffected, as did the fertility of accepted semen batches evaluated by the 60-day non-return rate.

Table 3. Sperm morphology in young bulls in October and December 1998 (n = 29) and in previous years (n = 103) at the same AI station.

	Previous years	October 1998	December 1998
Normal spermatozoa (%)	84.0 ± 9.1	71.0 ± 13.6	77.3 ± 14.4
Major sperm defects(%)	8.3 ± 4.3	19.5 ± 11.0	13.8 ± 9.6
Data presented as mean SD. All values within a row differ significantly (P < 0.01).			

5.19 EFFECT OF ACUTE BRSV INFECTION (III)

At the AI station, 54 out of the 79 young bulls had positive BRSV antibody titers at the age of 14 months. In general, either all or 0-2 of the young bulls in a quarantine group became infected based on seropositivity to BRSV. Of the randomly sampled 68 older bulls at the AI stations, 59 had negative BRSV antibody titers, and only 9 old bulls were seropositive.

The NR% differed significantly (P = 0.014) between BRSV seronegative and seropositive young bulls, being 76.9% and 75.2%, respectively. Bulls at Station 1 showed better fertility; overall NR% was 76.7% vs. NR% 75.4% for bulls at Station 2. However, the negative influence of BRSV infection on NR% was similar at both AI stations. Other factors in the statistical ANOVA model having an effect on NR% were insemination number (first vs.

later inseminations), parity (heifers vs. cows) and season (month of insemination) as well as interactions of station by BRSV and insemination month by BRSV.

Sperm morphology in BRSV-negative bulls was significantly better than in seropositive animals, the proportions of normal spermatozoa being 81.2% and 74.1%, respectively (P = 0.035). All classes of morphological abnormality were slightly elevated, although not significantly.

5.19 COMPARISON OF TWO INSEMINATION DOSES AND EFFECT OF MORPHOLOGY (IV)

The non-return rate in the 96 boars using the normal insemination dose of 3×10^9 spermatozoa (group B) was 84.0% compared with 75.8% in the 50 boars using a dose of 2×10^9 spermatozoa (group A) (P < 0.001). The corresponding size for primiparous litters was 10.7 versus 10.1 piglets (P < 0.001), and for multiparous litters 12.1 versus 11.7 piglets (P < 0.001). The results are summarized in Table 4.

When comparing those boars having ≥ 70% morphologically normal spermatozoa, the non-return rate in the 84 boars used with the normal insemination dose of 3×10^9 spermatozoa was 84.3% compared with 77.7% in the 46 boars using a dose of 2×10^9 spermatozoa (P < 0.001). The corresponding litter size for primiparous litters was 10.7 versus 10.2 piglets (P < 0.001), and for multiparous litters 12.2 versus 11.8 piglets (P < 0.001).

With the smaller insemination dose (group A), sperm morphology (percentage of normal spermatozoa) and all three fertility parameters were strongly correlated in the whole dataset (P < 0.01). For group B (normal insemination dose), the percentage of normal spermatozoa correlated with NR% (R = 0.223, P < 0.05), but there was no correlation with litter size.

When only the boars with more than 70% normal spermatozoa were included there were no correlations between the percentage of normal spermatozoa and any of the three fertility parameters, regardless of insemination dose. However, the negative correlation between the percentage of major sperm defects and litter size of multiparous farrowings remained significant, although the poorest boars by sperm morphology were excluded.

Table 4 Summary of boar semen and fertility parameters, presented as means SD.

	Group A (2 x 109)	Group B (3 x 109)	P
Non-return rate%	75.8 ± 8.8	84.0 ± 3.7	<0.001
Litter size of primiparous farrowings	10.1 ± 1.0	10.7 ± 0.6	<0.001
Litter size of primiparous farrowings	11.7 ± 0.7	12.1 ± 0.6	<0.001
Normal spermatozoa %	85.6 ± 15.3	85.2 ± 13.1	
Major sperm defects%	9.9 ± 14.7	5.5 ± 6.1	
Major sperm defects	4.4 ± 4.5	9.4 ± 10.9	

5.20 INTRAUTERINE (TRANSCERVICAL) INSEMINATION (V)

The intrauterine AI catheter was successfully passed through the cervix in 157 / 160 of the females (98.1%) at least at the second attempt (9.5%). Inserting the inner catheter took an extra minute. However, infusion of the AI dose was more rapid in the intrauterine AI so that for the whole insemination procedure, the intrauterine AI lasted for only an average of 22 seconds longer than the traditional AI. No blood was detectable on the uterine AI catheter after performing the AI.

Overall, live-born litter size was 11.3 ± 2.9, repeat breeding rate 4.2% and farrowing rate 91.2%. In the intrauterine insemination group, 93.6% of inseminated sows farrowed, whereas farrowing rate for the conventional insemination group was 88.8% (P = 0.13). Intrauterine insemination with a standard AI dose did not result in a significant improvement in the live-born litter size (11.5 ± 2.8 and 11.1 ± 3.0, respectively, P = 0.13).

The preceding satellite herd had a highly significant effect on the live-born litter size (12.4 ± 2.6; 11.1 ± 2.9; 10.8 ± 2.9 and 10.9 ± 2.9 for the four satellite herds, P < 0.01).

5.21 GENERAL DISCUSSION

AI is a reproductive technology that has made possible the effective use of best males, thus greatly improving the genetic quality of breeding herds. A prerequisite for the optimal use of this genetic material is to obtain acceptable fertility after AI. At high sperm numbers per AI dose bulls differ in their maximal NR%. That is unrelated to the rate at which they approach this. Therefore, screening of the semen for normality and evaluation of fertility is essential both to farmers and the AI industry.

For this thesis different aspects of semen quality and its evaluation were studied. Furthermore, the ultimate outcome of fertility, production of offspring, was the end-point in all five research projects included in this thesis.

5.22 SEMEN EVALUATION/FLUOROMETRIC METHOD

The fluorometric plasma membrane integrity assay (I) provided additional information to the routinely used sperm concentration and subjective motility evaluation in semen screening at AI stations. The new method was considered simple, objective, and rapid, and suitable for quality control. However, it was not effective in rejection of ejaculates in daily semen production because the regression between the percentage of viable spermatozoa and field fertility was negligible. The reasons might be the pre-selection of the semen which reduces the variability among ejaculates used, or the relatively high number of spermatozoa per insemination dose that may mask their functional weaknesses, so-called compensable deficiencies.

The correlation between sperm viability after thawing and fertility was demonstrated earlier. However, calculation of fluorescent cells in the microscope is time consuming, subjective and less accurate, and therefore not suitable for routine assays of high numbers of samples. Fluorometric plasma membrane integrity measurements provide a rapid and easy alternative for semen quality control. However, after our study, the increased cost-effectiveness of a newly launched flow cytometer in semen evaluation has made it the method of choice in many sperm laboratories.

5.23 TRICHOTHECENES

The decrease in semen quality caused by trichothecene mycotoxins (II) was manifested as impairment of initial and post-thaw progressive motility. The impairment began gradually 1.5 to 2 months after ingestion, and probably also inhalation, of moldy hay, and the semen remained of low quality for about five months after the end of feeding with moldy hay. The lowest semen quality (lowest proportion of ejaculates accepted for use in AI) was observed in December 1998, i.e., about two months after the cessation of this feeding. These findings indicate that the mycotoxins in the hay may have increased during storage, and that they exert their main effects at an early stage of spermatogenesis that takes approximately 62 days.

Epoxytrichothecenes, like T-2 and HT-2 toxins, inhibit protein as well as DNA and RNA synthesis, injuring organs with rapidly dividing cell populations such as germinal epithelium in testis (Ueno et al. 1984). Furthermore, T-2 is a potent inducer of apoptosis. T-2 inhibited testosterone synthesis and secretion in gerbils and guinea pigs, and induced degeneration and necrosis of spermatogenic cells in the semiferous tubules.

Ruminants are generally less susceptible to trichothecene mycotoxicosis than monogastric animals. The metabolism of ingested material by the ruminal microbes may be considered as a first line of defense against toxic materials present in the diet. On the other hand, ruminants may be at a disadvantage if substances become toxic as a result of the action of ruminal microbes. Another characteristic of trichothecene toxicity is the high susceptibility of animals, when exposed via the inhalation route, probably because of passing by the intestinal biodegradation/defense mechanisms.

The concentration of HT-2 toxin (570 ng / g) was markedly high in the hay as measured in both chemical and immunochemical assays. For comparison, found HT[-2] in the concentration range 10-20 ng / g in Finnish cereal samples. The daily amount of ingested mycotoxin certainly varied as a result of the probable uneven distribution of toxins in the hay.

Mycotoxins such as diacetoxyscirpenol, aflatoxin B1, zearalenone, and ochratoxin A have been blamed for deterioration of semen quality, for example, increased abnormalities in sperm morphology and decrease in motility. Fenske and Fink-Gremmels (1990) reported that T-2 inhibits testosterone secretion *in vitro*. However, HT-2 and T-2 toxins have not earlier been implicated in impairment of semen quality *in vivo*. The effects of low trichothecene contents on testicular function and spermatozoa remain to be fully evaluated in an experimental design.

5.24 BRSV

BRSV is often underestimated in animals older than 6 months, but our results (III) clearly show the influence of BRSV epizootics on sperm quality and field fertility in young AI bulls. Despite the usually mild disease in older animals, it may cause economic losses to farmers and AI organizations due to sub-fertility and need for early culling of bulls.

The mode of transmission in natural infection has not been confirmed, but direct contact is probably necessary. Available data to date do not allow conclusions to be drawn on the length of shedding of the virus and investigations are lacking on the length of quarantine required to avoid transmission to susceptible animals. However, quarantine of young bulls proved to be effective; at the AI stations none of the mature bulls fell ill or showed any decline in semen quality, and almost all remained seronegative for BRSV. It is not known exactly how long antibodies against BRSV remain in sera of adult cattle, but it is months or even years without re-infection, confirming the disease-free status of older bulls.

BRSV infection in young (6-12 months old) bulls seems to increase testicular fibrosis (Barth et al. 2008) by an unknown mechanism that might have some immunological background, similar to the pathological changes in lungs caused by the BRS virus where fibrosis is common. Barth et al. (2008) suggested that during the active process leading to fibrosis of the testicular tissue, spermatogenesis is adversely affected, and this is later seen as poor sperm morphology. This is in accordance with our findings during and after BRSV epizootics. The old bulls instead, having had BRSV infection long ago but being still seropositive, had normal sperm morphology, as expected, since no ongoing harmful process or acute infection affected sperm production in testicles, contrary to the case of young BRSV infected bulls.

5.25 SEASONALITY

Although often suspected, it became clear from these studies (I-V) that both cows and sows still show a tendency to be seasonal breeders despite domestication and active breeding. There were seasons with lowered fertility, although not total infertility. This phenomenon was earlier described for sows in Finland, and for cows in Norway, where a marked heat stress during the summer months is not a problem/confounding factor. The seasonal effect in reproduction has been shown to be caused by variation in day length and mediated by melatonin.

5.26 THE EFFECT OF SPERM MORPHOLOGY AND INSEMINATION DOSE

The importance of normal sperm morphology in bulls, goats, stallions and men is well known. These studies confirm the significance of sperm morphology also in AI bulls and boars; earlier studies with this pre-selected material have been somewhat controversial. The controversy might be explained by the quite high numbers of sperm that are often used for insemination, even though we were able to find the effect also with higher sperm numbers (IV) in accordance with Saacke (2008). However, sperm morphology is not sensitive enough to rank males within "normal" limits for fertility.

The effect of poor semen morphology is multiplied when the insemination dose decreases and otherwise compensable morphological deficiencies can no longer be overcome. This leads to decreased fertility rates and litter sizes in pluriparous animals. The recommended total sperm count in an insemination dose ranges from 1.5 or 2 x 109 to 6 x 109 for boars. With the routinely used insemination dose of 3 x 109, the number of spermatozoa is not a limiting factor and field trials may not detect small differences, which agrees with our results (IV). Some characteristics of spermatozoa, including chromosomal aberrations, DNA damage or aberrant chromatin structure, cannot be compensated for by increasing the number of spermatozoa, but affect the pregnancy rate and litter size at all insemination doses. Other characteristics (most classical parameters) of spermatozoa affect their ability to reach and fertilize oocytes, and the increasing number of spermatozoa in the insemination dose can therefore improve the chances of success. The morphological classification introduced by Blom (1983) is well suited for practical purposes to detect different sperm populations in a sample, not only in bulls, but also in horses and boars, allowing its use to determine an optimal insemination dose for a male.

Conducting a semen morphology examination once before entering boars into AI use, as suggested by Larsson et al. (1980), proved to be beneficial in predicting the suitability of a young boar for breeding (IV). In the case of adult boars, repeated examinations are recommended, but the optimal examination frequency remains unclear. This applies to AI bulls as well. Semen morphology has a limited positive predictive value for field fertility, especially in pre-selected (for motility, concentration) samples. It does, however, help to screen-out overtly poor-quality ejaculates. It is quite easy and inexpensive to perform, not only in a reference laboratory, but also in AI stations, although it requires some experience.

5.27 INTRAUTERINE INSEMINATION IN SOWS

With the standard insemination dose of 3 x 109 spermatozoa, both litter size and farrowing rate in sows were unaffected by intrauterine insemination (V), so the method did not lead to a significant improvement of fertility using such a high dose. As reported a slight reduction in fertility using intrauterine AI with 1×10^9 spermatozoa / dose compared with 2 or 3×10^9 spermatozoa / dose. We did not compare the effect on fertility of smaller insemination doses, but at least when using 3×10^9 spermatozoa, no additional benefit ensued in comparison with traditional AI.

The duration of insertion of the uterine AI catheter was only slightly longer than with the traditional method, as reported earlier. Simultaneously, we also observed that the time to dispose the AI dose was shorter with the intrauterine than with the traditional catheter, so that the whole AI procedure lasted only 22 seconds longer using the intrauterine catheter. In principle, insertion of the inner catheter through the cervix, in addition to the traditional AI catheter, may provide additional cervical stimulation that appears to induce further myometrial contractility. This may explain the faster infusion time of the uterine AI dose found in the present study.

The uterine AI seems to be a practical and feasible method of inseminating the sow and the time required to pass the cervix with the catheter appears not to be a major obstacle either. It might be most profitable when maximizing the use of the superior boars.

6

ARTIFICIAL INSEMINATION AND EMBRYO TRANSFER IN GOATS

6.1 INTRODUCTION

- Artificial insemination (AI) is a key technology that can be used for improving animal production. Through consistent use of AI, herd genetics can be advanced at a rapid rate using semen from sires selected based on expected progeny differences (EPDs) or selection indexes targeted to improve various traits including weaning weights, growth rates, slaughter weights, milk production, physical type as well as maternal longevity and production efficiency. Introduction

  Effective estrus synchronization, ovulation synchronization and transcervical insemination methods for AI are now available to goat producers and can be used to increase the efficiency of herd reproductive management. In addition, for producers with high-quality genetic stock or those who want to rapidly change the genetics of their herds, the use of embryo transfer will facilitate attainment of these objectives. Successful implementation of any of these reproductive management technologies, however, requires careful attention to protocol specifics, record-keeping and doe management.

  of AI to the US dairy cattle industry, coupled with essentially universal acceptance of computerized dairy records management systems, revolutionized the domestic dairy industry such that today the US dairy herd is at its lowest number of cows yet greatest production per animal in history, effectively supplying milk for the largest population in US history. More recently, swine producers have also recognized the significant advantages of implementing AI to advance animal production programs within their industry.

- While AI is a technology that enables the dissemination of selected male genetics, embryo transfer (ET) is a technology that enables the dissemination of selected female genetics. In this way, productive genes carried by dams can be more rapidly spread within a population by having less valuable dams carrying offspring of elite females instead. In addition, through the use of ET, frozen embryos can be moved around the world more easily and safely compared to movement of postnatal animals.

⊙ Utilization of either AI or ET requires careful doe management and is most effective when these technologies are used in conjunction with estrus or ovulation synchronization. Synchronization allows groups of does to be managed together, focusing labor needs and reducing time input. Therefore, this paper will address the topics of estrus and ovulation synchronization, artificial insemination and embryo transfer in goats focusing on practical application of these technologies for herd improvement with particular emphasis on synchronization and AI. Discussion will be limited to application of these technologies during the normal breeding season rather than for breeding management during the anestrous season.

⊙ Artificial insemination (AI) is an important technology for improving animal production. Through consistent use of AI, herd genetics can be advanced at a rapid rate. While AI is a technology that enables the dissemination of selected male genetics, embryo transfer (ET) is a technology that enables the dissemination of selected female genetics and, by using ET, frozen embryos can be moved around the world at significantly reduced costs compared to movement of adult animals. Utilization of either AI or ET requires careful doe management and is most effective when these technologies are used in conjunction with estrus or ovulation synchronization. This paper will address the topics of estrus and ovulation synchronization, artificial insemination and embryo transfer in goats with a focus on the practical application of synchronization and AI for herd improvement.

6.2 ESTRUS SYNCHRONIZATION

The goal of any synchronization program is to group animals so they enter into the same physiological state as simultaneously as possible. In the case of estrus synchronization, the goal is to have does in heat as close to the same time as possible, allowing animals to be heat checked as a group with individual does bred after they show estrus. Labor efforts are highly focused allowing one to take advantage of AI for breeding. In practice, most methods for estrus synchronization result in a group of does coming into estrus over about a 48 h period, requiring both morning and evening heat checks before, during and after this targeted time interval. When using AI, does found in estrus are bred 12 h after they are first detected in heat by the AM-PM rule; that is, if a doe is found in heat in the morning, she would be bred that evening and if in heat in the evening, she would be bred the following morning.

⊙ A number of useful methods are available to producers for estrus synchronization in goats during the breeding season. These include progesterone-based or prostaglandin-based protocols as well as combined methods utilizing both progesterone- and prostaglandin-based treatments.

6.2.1 Progesterone-Based Synchronization

Progesterone-based synchronization consists of treatments with either the natural hormone, progesterone, or with synthetic derivatives of progesterone known as progestogens. As an example, natural progesterone can be found in a controlled intravaginal drug releasing device (CIDR, Pfizer Inc.) (Rathbone, et al, 1998). Examples of progestogens include melengestrol acetate (MGA), altrenogest or norgestomet. These agents mimic the action of the corpus luteum (CL), a progesterone-secreting structure located on the ovary. If a doe has a CL that is secreting progesterone, she will not show estrus. The CL also functions to maintain pregnancy, if the doe has been bred successfully. Whether using the natural hormone or a progestogen, similar physiological responses occur within the animal. However, differences exist between the various progestogens with regard to routes of administration, dosages required, effectiveness and cost.

- ◉ Because CIDRs are commercially available and simple to use for most producers, the remainder of this discussion will focus on natural progesterone-based synchronization using CIDRs. Treatment consists of a single CIDR being gently inserted into a doe's vaginal vault with the device remaining in place for varying periods until removed. Elevated levels of progesterone released by the CIDR prevent the doe from coming into estrus until the device is removed. After CIDR removal, the doe will come into heat about 36-72 h later and can be bred by AI. CIDRs can be administered for varying periods, typically ranging from 9 to 21 days. Any does not settled after AI at the first estrus following CIDR removal will remain synchronized for the second estrus 3 weeks later.

- ◉ Retention rates for CIDRs in goats are about 90%. In general, these devices work well with females of moderate to large frame size. Doelings or adult does of smaller frame breeds may have difficulty accommodating the size of the CIDR in their reproductive tracts. CIDRs can be purchased from commercial animal health and livestock suppliers and do not require a prescription. However, because CIDRs are only approved for use in sheep in the United States, their use in goats would be considered extra-label.

6.2.2 Prostaglandin-Based Synchronization

Prostaglandin F2alpha (PGF) is a naturally occurring hormone that can be used to bring females into estrus. It is effective only if females are normally cycling and have a corpus luteum (CL) present on their ovaries. The CL is the ovarian structure that produces progesterone in the female, keeping her out of estrus. In a normal estrous cycle, secretion of PGF from the uterus destroys the CL and the doe comes into heat.

PGF is marketed as the product dinoprost (Lutalyse, Pfizer, Inc.). To obtain PGF, or any of its synthetic analogs, a prescription is required from your veterinarian. Synchronization with PGF typically involves administration of 2 treatments, with the first given on Day 1 and the second on Day 10. Lutalyse dosages can vary from 7.5mg to 15mg per injection. In our experience, the 15 mg dosage provides consistent and reliable results (Bowdridge, et al, 2013). However, lower doses can also be effective. Does will come into heat after either the first or second injection and can be bred by AI at either time. To better conserve labor, animals are usually not heat checked after the first injection but only after the second PGF injection. Eighty to 90% of the treated does will show estrus 36-96 h after the second PGF injection. Animals can be bred by AI using the AM-PM rule. There is no decrease in fertility at the synchronized estrus when PGF is used.

6.2.3 Combined CIDR and PGF Synchronization

Effective protocols for estrus synchronization in goats can also involve the use to both CIDRs and PGF. Use of a combined protocol can alleviate the fertility depression associated with longer term CIDR use, resulting in good synchronization and fertility at the estrus immediately post-treatment. A relatively simple combined CIDR-PGF protocol involves a short, 6-day CIDR treatment. A CIDR is inserted on Day 1 in the morning and six days later is removed (am or pm on Day 6). An injection of PGF must be given either at the time of CIDR insertion or CIDR removal. If PGF is given at the time of CIDR removal, does will come into estrus 36-72 h later and can be bred by AI based on estrus detection and the AM/PM rule.

6.2.4 Use of Bucks to Breed Synchronized Females

Although producers will make the greatest genetic gains coupling estrus synchronization protocols with AI, it is important to note that estrus synchronization can also be combined with natural breeding. Use of estrus synchronization in this context allows producers to take advantage of grouping females for their breeding and subsequent kidding periods, making overall reproductive management of the doe herd more predictable. Although few studies exist that have evaluated buck to doe ratios when females have been estrus synchronized, based on studies in cattle, it is recommended that only mature males be used for this purpose. A mature buck can be expected to handle ratios of 1:15-20 synchronized females with good pregnancy rates to the synchronized estrus.

6.2.5 Ovulation Synchronization

Ovulation synchronization, as its name implies, is a method that allows producers to synchronize the release of the egg from the ovary, rather than simply synchronizing the female's estrus behavior. The major advantage of ovulation synchronization is that a producer does not need to perform any heat checking of their does prior to breeding. Rather than relying on detection of estrus behavior that is frequently challenging to reliably determine in does, ovulation is synchronized and the females are bred by AI at a fixed time during the treatment protocol. This is referred to as "timed AI" or TAI. Ovulation synchronization further focuses labor needs to the preselected day of breeding only because heat checking is not used and breeding dates can be precisely scheduled in advance of the breeding season. Pregnancy rates following ovulation synchronization with TAI using a single dose of frozen semen are comparable to those obtained for AI breed-by-estrus protocols.

Successful ovulation synchronization-TAI protocols have been developed for goats. These protocols utilize several different hormones in sequence to control CL function, stimulate follicular development and regulate ovulation. Progesterone-free protocols are also available and utilize treatment combinations of PGF and the ovulatory hormone, gonadotropin releasing hormone (GnRH), to induce a synchronized ovulation in preparation for TAI.

Over the past five breeding seasons, we have evaluated pregnancy and kidding rates achieved following three different ovulation synchronization- TAI protocols compared to rates achieved by breed-by-estrus AI controls. Timelines for each of the ovulation synchronization-TAI protocols examined are illustrated in Figure 1. In these studies, does were assigned to receive either the NC.Synch, CIDR.6, CIDR.11 or Control treatments. Does in the NC.Synch, CIDR.6 and CIDR.11 groups were bred by TAI whereas does in the Control group were bred by AI-based heat checking and the AM-PM rule. All treatments were scheduled to begin in the morning on any treatment day. All inseminations were performed by experienced inseminators using the NCSU simplified catheter-based transcervical method (see below) with a single dose of frozen semen. Pregnancy rates were based on detection by transabdominal ultrasonography at 55 and 85 days post-insemination. Because not all treatments were represented each year, the number of does in each of the treatment groups varied (Figure 2).

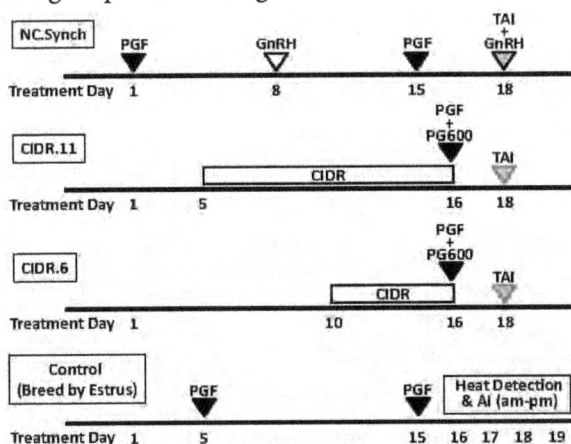

Fig. 1: Ovulation (NC.Synch, CIDR.11, CIDR.6) or estrus (Control) synchronization protocols evaluated in the NCSU goat herd between 2007 and 2012.

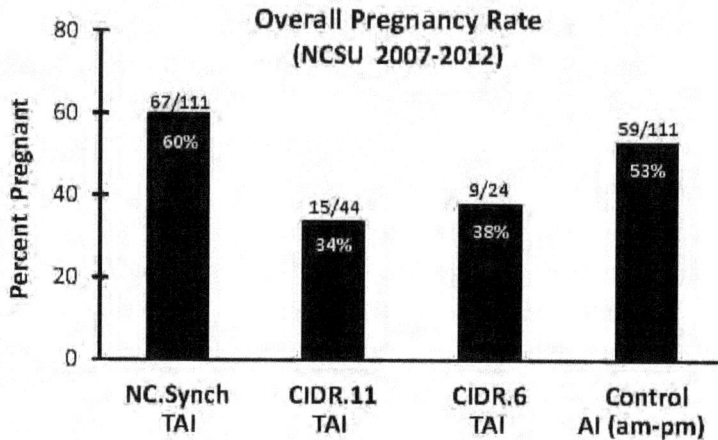

Fig. 2: Pregnancy rates for ovulation or estrus synchronization protocols evaluated in the NCSU goat herd between 2007 and 2012.

The pregnancy rate following the NC.Synch-TAI treatment was comparable to the rate for the breed-by-estrus AI control ($p = 0.28$). In contrast, pregnancy rates were significantly ($p < 0.01$) lower in the CIDR.6-TAI and CIDR.11-TAI groups compared to NC.Synch-TAI. These data demonstrate that satisfactory pregnancy rates can be achieved with a single dose of frozen semen using NC.Synch-TAI protocol. Furthermore, use of an ovulation synchronization protocol eliminates the need for heat checking before AI and allows breeding to occur on a schedule that can be set by the producer while still maintaining pregnancy rates comparable to the traditional breed-by-estrus method. Use of PG600 in the experiments described above provided a source of the hormone, equine chorionic gonadotropin (eCG), to induce additional ovarian stimulation, potentially increasing the number of kids produced. Repeated use of this hormone in goats, either within a breeding season or across breeding seasons is not recommended. Like cattle, goats will develop antibodies against this hormone, usually after two eCG administrations, making females permanently resistant to its effects. Use of the NC. Synch-TAI method during the breeding season eliminates the need for eCG treatment, does not involve the use of CIDRs and is a very simple ovulation synchronization protocol for producers to follow. It can only be used during the breeding season when does are naturally cycling, however. Veterinary prescriptions are required to obtain the hormones used in this protocol.

6.3 ARTIFICIAL INSEMINATION (AI)

There are two basic techniques used for AI in goats, laparoscopic insemination and transcervical insemination. Pregnancy rates are generally higher for laparoscopic insemination compared to transcervical insemination. However, laparoscopic insemination requires highly skilled inseminators, typically veterinarians or individuals under veterinary supervision, because minor surgical procedures and application of anesthesia is required. In contrast, transcervical insemination techniques can be learned and performed by the producer and do not require surgical entry into the animal or application of anesthesia.

6.3.1 Laparscopic Insemination

Laparoscopic insemination involves a limited surgical entry into the abdominal portion of the body cavity of the doe with guided injection of the semen dose directly into each uterine horn. It is typically performed by trained veterinarians and veterinary assistants skilled in the technique. Briefly, for laparoscopic insemination, the doe is anesthetized and placed on a surgical table in dorsal recumbency with her rear quarters elevated above her head. Portions of the abdominal area of her belly are scrubbed and small incisions are made on either side of the midline. Sterile instruments are introduced into each incision and the abdominal cavity inflated with carbon dioxide or sterile air to facilitate visualization of the uterus and ovaries. Insemination is accomplished by visualization of each uterine horn using a laparoscope and deposition of semen into the uterine lumen using a sterile insemination needle. Once the doe is anesthetized, the entire insemination procedure takes about 5-10 minutes. Following insemination, the incisions are sutured and the doe is returned to a recovery pen where she will recover in about 10 minutes.

Pregnancy rates achieved with laparoscopic insemination are approximately 60-80%, making use of this technique an attractive option for producers with large numbers of animals requiring insemination. In contrast, this option may not be cost-effective for producers with fewer animals. Use of ovulation synchronization and TAI protocols, however, can make laparoscopic insemination a more attractive option even for smaller producers because specific insemination dates can be conveniently prearranged.

6.3.2 Transcervical Insemination

The cervix of the doe has 4 tightly closed, cartilaginous rings that provide structure to the cervix and, along with cervical mucus, form a protective physical barrier against the entry of foreign particles. To achieve the highest pregnancy rates for AI, semen must be deposited into the uterine body or into each of the uterine horns. Deposition of semen into the uterus requires that all 4 cervical rings must be passed during the insemination procedure. The small size of the doe's reproductive tract, particularly for nulliparous (virgin) or young primiparous (once kidded) does, in addition to the tightness of the cervical rings and their typical lack of alignment can make passing the insemination rod during transcervical AI a challenging task. However, several methods for transcervical insemination have been developed and are available, some of which are similar to procedures described for nonsurgical embryo transfer in goats.

6.3.3 Standard AI Method (Tube speculum)

The simplest transcervical AI method involves the use of a tube-like speculum and a standard French-style insemination gun. The speculum, with a detachable light, is inserted into the vaginal vault of the doe and used to visualize the external cervical os which is the entry point into the cervical channel. Frozen semen is available in 1/4cc or 1/2cc straws and must be appropriately thawed prior to use. Once the semen straw is prepared and placed into the insemination gun, a clean sheath is overlaid to protect the semen and reduce cross-contamination between does. Sheaths can have either standard (rounded) or apex (pointed) ends that can aid in achieving deeper penetration of the cervix. The insemination gun is introduced through the speculum and the inseminator attempts to pass the insemination gun through the cervix and deposit the semen into the uterine body. Following insemination, the gun and speculum are removed and the speculum disinfected between does. The single-use AI gun sheath is disposed of appropriately.

The major advantage of the standard method is that it is a simple and easily mastered technique that is reasonably effective with older, multiparous does. The major disadvantage of this technique is that it is difficult to pass the insemination gun through the small cervix of a young doe or through the cervix if it is highly convoluted. In many cases, use of the standard technique results in deposition of the semen in the cervix if all of the cervical rings cannot be passed. Under controlled conditions, pregnancy rates following the use of the standard technique are low, typically in the range of 20-30%.

6.3.4 Deep Cornual (Uterine) Insemination (Catheter-Within-Catheter) Method

In 2005, Sohnrey and Holtz reported the development of a novel method for transcervical insemination of goats. In their method, semen is deposited deep into the uterine horn (cornua) by means of a catheter-within-catheter technique. This technique relies on use of a soft, small diameter pediatric urinary catheter stiffened with an insemination gun stylet to gain entry into the uterine body and individual uterine horn. To facilitate passage through the cervix, the doe's hindquarters are raised and a Pozzi tenaculum forceps is used to grasp the cervix and align the cervical rings. Once the catheter is positioned into the uterine horn, the stylet is removed and a small diameter insemination tubing is threaded through the urinary catheter and used to deposit fresh or frozen-thawed semen into the upper portion of the uterine horn. The urinary catheter is then repositioned into the opposite uterine horn and the second half of the semen sample is deposited deep into that horn to complete the insemination. With trained technicians, the entire procedure takes about 5-10 min and does not involve any surgical entry or anesthesia of the doe. Furthermore, pregnancy rates following deep cornual insemination were greater than those for laparoscopic insemination in their study. In a subsequent study, pregnancy rates using ovulation synchronization with TAI of a single dose of frozen semen were 58% and kidding rates similar at 53%. These pregnancy rates are comparable to those obtained for beef cattle for first-service insemination after TAI using frozen semen.

6.3.5 NCSU Simplified Catheter-Based Method

At North Carolina State University, a modified insemination technique was developed (Farin and Knox, unpublished) based on the deep uterine technique reported by Sohnrey and Holtz (2005) and the nonsurgical embryo transfer technique described by Kraemer (1989). This technique relies on use of the pediatric urinary catheter, insemination gun stylet and Pozzi tenaculum forceps as described to gain passage through the cervix and entry into the uterine body. In the NCSU method, the tip of the catheter is placed in the uterine body, with catheter position verified by digital palpation through the vaginal vault or by predetermined measurement. Once in position, the stylet is removed, a syringe barrel introduced onto the distal end of the pediatric catheter and the semen sample is deposited into the uterine body though the pediatric catheter itself. Once the semen is deposited into the uterine body, the catheter and Pozzi forceps are removed. With skilled technicians, the entire procedure takes about 5-8 min.

Pregnancy rates following estrus synchronization and AI or ovulation synchronization and TAI using the simplified catheter method for transcervical insemination are comparable (Figure 2) to those reported for the deep cornual insemination (catheter-within-catheter) method. Furthermore, pregnancy rates are greater for either of the catheter-based methods compared to the standard AI technique.

6.4 EMBRYO TRANSFER IN GOATS

Embryo transfer (ET) is a reproductive technology that allows producers to take advantage of high-quality genetics in their dams. In addition, ET can be used to rapidly introduce new genetic lines or entirely new breeds into existing herds. For the successful application of ET within a goat herd, intensive reproductive management and excellent record-keeping is required. In addition, careful analysis of cost-benefit ratios must be considered before an ET program is started. Kids must be highly marketable or of high genetic value to balance the costs associated with developing an ET program.

The basic steps in the ET process are illustrated in Figure 3. Donor females of high genetic quality are superovulated with hormonal treatments that cause them to ovulate more than the normal number of eggs. The donor doe is inseminated with semen from a genetically desirable sire and the fertilized embryos are allowed to grow within the donor's reproductive tract for approximately 1 week. After this period, the embryos are recovered from the uterus of the donor female by uterine lavage (flushing). The recovered embryos are identified, assessed and from 1 to 3 embryos are transferred into the uterus of a recipient female that is of lower genetic quality and whose reproductive cycle has been carefully synchronized to match the cycle of the donor female. In this way, embryos are transferred from the uterus of the original donor into a uterus at the same gestational stage within the recipient female, and thus, can continue development to term unaffected. After an appropriate rest period (2-3 months), the process can be repeated with the original donor female who would be superovulated and bred again to produce more embryos for transfer. Because protocols for freezing goat embryos are available, it is also feasible for recovered embryos to be frozen and held for transfer at a later date.

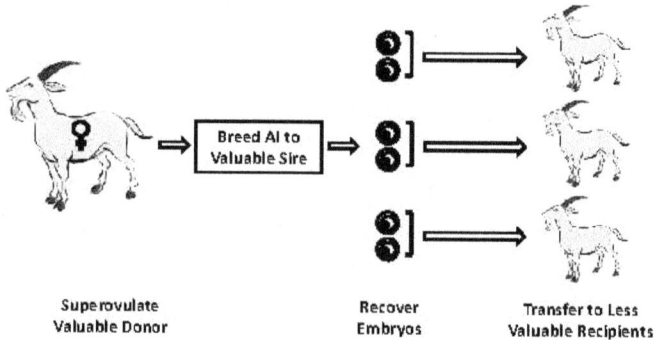

Fig. 3: Overview of the embryo transfer process for goats.

Although ET in cattle is performed entirely with transcervical (nonsurgical) procedures, ET in goats is performed using either laparotomy (abdominal surgery) or, more frequently, laparoscopy for embryo recovery coupled with laparoscopy for transfer of the recovered embryos into the recipient female. Nonsurgical procedures for embryo recovery in goats have been reported. However, most donor flushes in goats are still performed using laparoscopic recovery. Producers considering an ET program for their herd must arrange to work with a veterinarian highly experienced in these techniques to have these procedures performed on farm.

Implementation of a successful ET program requires effective donor and recipient management. To successfully produce sufficient numbers of embryos of desired genetics for recovery, donor females are estrus synchronized, superovulated and bred by AI. Successful superovuation protocols for goats have been published and entail a combination of CIDR treatment, PGF or PGF-analog injection, follicle stimulating hormone (FSH) treatment to induce follicular development and GnRH treatment to induce ovulation. An example of a donor treatment schedule is illustrated in Figure 4.

Using either laparoscopy or nonsurgical embryo recovery, between 0 and 18 embryos are produced per donor, with about 4-6 on average. It is important to note that superovulation is not a well-controlled phenomenon and, based on data in cattle, about 25% of donor cow flushes do not produce any embryos whereas about 25% of donor cow flushes produce an excessive number of embryos. Therefore, when using ET, it is often suggested that at least 3-4 donor females be set up for a specific ET session and that the producer should expect, *on average*, about 4-6 embryos to be produced per donor per session.

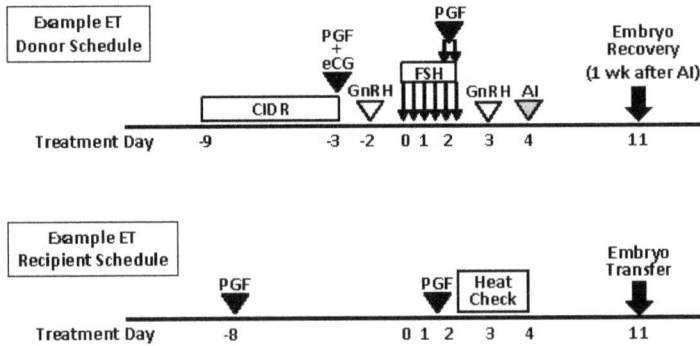

Fig. 4: Example donor superovulation and recipient estrus synchronization treatment schedules for embryo transfer in goats.

In conjunction with donor preparation, the recipient females also need to be estrus synchronized so that they are at the same stage of the estrous cycle as the donor females. Recipient does are heat checked so the first day of their cycle is known, but they are not bred so that they do not have embryos of their own in their reproductive tract. Recipient cycles can be synchronized by a variety of estrus or ovulation synchronization protocols, an example of which is illustrated in Figure 4. Embryo transfers are done by laparoscopy with 1-3 embryos transferred into the recipient female's uterus. A good rule of thumb for estimating the number of recipient females needed for an ET session is to have about 3-4 recipients synchronized for each donor doe scheduled to undergo embryo recovery. If extra embryos are produced and no additional recipients are available, embryos can be frozen and stored for future transfer. Furthermore, if frozen embryos are obtained by the producer, recipient does can be synchronized, heat checked and 1-3 embryos transferred into the recipient's uterus by laparoscopy at an appropriate time convenient for the producer and veterinarian.

7

CANINE ARTIFICIAL INSEMINATION

7.1 INTRODUCTION: AN OVERVIEW

Artificial insemination is an assisted reproductive technique that can be used to compensate for some causes of canine infertility. Many reasons may lead to the request for artificial insemination in dogs. In most cases, inability or unwillingness to copulate naturally or difficulty in achieving or maintaining a successful pregnancy is involved in the decision to seek help. Assisted reproduction in bitches that do not cycle or that have abnormal cycle patterns presents a different challenge.

Artificial insemination is an imitation of the natural act of mating. It involves instillation of semen removed from a male dog into the cranial vagina or uterus of a bitch during the most fertile time of her estrous cycle. It is most frequently indicated in bitches that have normal estrous cycles but have a history of failure to conceive after natural mating or inability to be bred naturally. Successful artificial insemination results in pregnancy.

Coordination is key to increasing the probability of obtaining a successful pregnancy through artificial insemination. Although time-consuming, well-coordinated efforts are more likely to be rewarded with success. Without thorough planning, artificial insemination may be a frustrating exercise. Preexamination of the proposed dam and sire is needed to determine infectious, metabolic, or genetic defects that could lead to potential spread of infectious disease, failure to conceive, or early termination of pregnancy. Ovulation timing should be used to determine when the bitch is most fertile, especially when shipping chilled semen or when using frozen semen, if only one insemination is possible. Knowledge of the semen preparation used is important in order to determine the appropriate insemination method.

7.2 PREBREEDING CONCERNS

7.2.1 Physical Examination

⊙ Ensuring that both the dam and sire are healthy is important. The general health of the dam and sire is assessed with a breeding soundness and prebreeding examination, respectively.[2-5] Only healthy animals without heritable genetic defects should be considered for artificial insemination. Information concerning possible heritable diseases should be obtained by questioning the owner. A general physical examination of the dam should be performed before, not at the time of, insemination to identify any problems. Likewise, the sire's semen quality should be ascertained well in advance of the insemination procedure. Poor-quality semen may result in an unsuccessful pregnancy or contribute to small litter sizes.

⊙ Even with a healthy dam and sire, insemination may not be successful. The experience of the person performing the procedure and the difficulty of the technique used may influence the outcome. Coordination of ovulation in the bitch, semen acquisition from the desired stud dog, and insemination during the most fertile period of estrus is the most critical aspect of artificial insemination. Therefore, the owner should be made aware of every factor of artificial insemination before proceeding, including the time commitment and financial cost of the procedure. A checklist can be used as a guide to educate the owner. Although discouragement is not warranted, the owner must fully understand the process and be advised of the probability of success or failure.

7.2.2 Indications for Artificial Insemination

Males and Females

⊙ Inability or unwillingness to copulate naturally

⊙ Desired breeding partner in different location

⊙ Import and quarantine regulations

Males

⊙ Utilization of champion sire after death

⊙ Inability to breed naturally (e.g., stiffness or weak hindquarters caused by previous inJury or arthritis)

⊙ Prevention of overutilization of stud dog

Females

⊙ Congenital or acquired vaginal anomalies

⊙ Subfertile due tot age or previous scar tissue form difficulty whelpuing

7.2.3 Estrus and Ovulation

The estrous cycle in bitches is divided into four stages: proestrus, estrus, diestrus (or metestrus), and anestrus. Artificial insemination is always performed during estrus because it is the stage when ovulation occurs. This is the most fertile time of the estrous cycle.1-3 Estrus can last from 3 to 21 days in bitches, but the average duration is 9 days.3,6 External signs and the behavior of the bitch during proestrus and estrus are related to hormonal changes.

During proestrus, follicle-stimulating hormone secreted by the pituitary gland induces the development and growth of ovarian follicles. The ovarian follicles secrete estrogen, and as estrogen levels increase, the vulva begins to swell and the uterus releases a sanguineous discharge. The swelling of the vulva is caused by swelling and proliferation of the vaginal mucosa. These changes can be seen via endoscopy as an increase in the height of the longitudinal vaginal folds. The vaginal epithelial cell type also changes in preparation for copulation; detection of this cell type on a vaginal smear indicates an increase in estrogen. The male dog becomes interested in the bitch as a result of pheromones that are secreted at this time. The bitch may seem interested in the male dog but is not receptive to mounting and intromission.

In early estrus, the ovarian follicles continue to grow and secrete estrogen. As estrus progresses, the estrogen levels begin to decline as the luteinized follicular cells begin to produce progesterone. In late estrus, declining estrogen levels and rising progesterone levels trigger the secretion of a high level of luteinizing hormone (LH) from the pituitary gland. Ovulation occurs 24 to 48 hours after this peak increase in LH. At this time, the vulva is turgid and less swollen. The uterine discharge becomes serosanguineous and decreases or completely stops. The predominant cell type of the vaginal mucosa changes again, the vaginal mucosa becomes less edematous, and the bitch becomes receptive to the dog.

Released oocytes cannot be fertilized immediately after ovulation, when they are at the beginning of the uterine tube. The most fertile days are 2 to 3 days after ovulation,[3,6] when the oocytes have descended through most of the uterine tube and are ready and available for fertilization. Natural mating or artificial insemination can be instituted during this 2- to 3-day period.

After ovulation, the remaining follicular cells develop into corpora lutea (yellow bodies) that continue to secrete progesterone. This continued rise in progesterone signals the onset of diestrus. In diestrus, there is another change in the primary cell type of the vaginal mucosa and no vulvar discharge. Vaginal and vulvar swelling decrease, the vulva gradually decreases in size, and the bitch again becomes nonreceptive to the dog.

7.3 METHODS OF OVULATION TIMING

5.3.1 Health Status Check Before Artificial Insemination

- ◉ Information About Dam and Sire
- ◉ Harilscrili. andocnulperrietztcaltrilvaetion sta., deworming,
- ◉ Hanisctioprryet=sg thillgpssy and surgeries with outcome

- Current drug therapy, environment, and Wet

- General physical examination with special attention to geWtal organs

- OrthopeWc Foundation for Animals certification for hip dysplasia for large-breed dogs; other certifications if needed; details of possible genetic diseases

- Serologic testing for Brucella

- Establishment of herpesvirus serologic state (positive or negative) Information About Dam Only (Prebreeding Examination)

- Details of past estrous cycles (especially last cycle before presentation)

- Details of past breedings) and whether it (they) resulted in pregnancy and whelping

- Details of past litters (e.g., litter size, health of puppies)

- History of and reason(s) for maternal and sibling infertility

- Digital vagnal exanlination, observation of vulvar conformation, palpation of mammary gancls

- Vaginal cytology

- Vaginoscopy (optional) Information About Sire Only (Breeding Soundness Examination) linesttaainsc:sf Vsotpbe rne ebtlhgeradfteerttese deirs1Pgr a" Y

- HoiltolreydoofghLrbvr:cf'ten semen is collected from the dog

- Examination of testicles, penis, and prostate gland

- Semen collection and results

- Ep=orLoifdsemen color and volume and pH of

- Semen analysis with sperm count, viability, cytology, and morphology

- Microbial culture of ejaculate (optional)

Ovulation timing is the determination of the most fertile days of estrus. Ovulation timing is used as part of the artificial insemination procedure to ensure that ova are present in the uterine tube at the time of the semen injection. An advantage of ovulation timing is that it allows the time of whelping to be determined exactly, which is especially important when a cesarean section is needed.

7.3.2 Vaginal Cytology

Vaginal cytology is the laboratory test most commonly used to confirm proestrus and estrus. For this test, a microscope slide is prepared from vaginal smears made by inserting a sterile cotton swab through the vulva into the vagina, avoiding the vestibule. A speculum or finger may be used to guard the swab on entry into the vagina. The cells from the cranial vagina walls easily exfoliate upon swabbing. After the cells are collected, the swab is rolled onto a glass microscope slide. The slide is allowed to air dry and is then stained, usually with a Diff-Quik stain, although other stains can also be used.

In proestrus, vaginal epithelial cells change from small parabasal cells with large nuclei to larger intermediate cells and then to very large cornified cells. The parabasal cells have basophilic blue-staining cytoplasm. The nuclei are easily seen, and the amount of nuclear material is roughly equal to the amount of cytoplasm. Intermediate cells are larger than the parabasal cells and less basophilic. The nuclei are smaller in comparison to the cytoplasm, and the cell borders are still somewhat rounded. Cornified cells have small or nonexistent nuclei and are large and square. High numbers of intermediate and cornified epithelial cells, red and white blood cells, and bacteria are evident during proestrus.

In estrus, the number of cornified cells increases. At the time of ovulation, the primary epithelial cell type seen on vaginal cytology is the cornified epithelial cell. The microscopic visualization of primarily (usually 90%) superficial epithelial cells and abundant bacteria without white blood cells indicates late estrus and probably ovulation.

The accuracy of vaginal cytology depends on the experience of the person(s) performing the swab, preparing the slide, and reading the slide. Therefore, it may be beneficial to use additional methods of determining ovulation to confirm the results of vaginal cytology.

7.3.3 Vaginoscopy

The hormone-related changes in the vaginal mucosa that take place during proestrus and estrus can be easily seen with the proper equipment and are consistent enough to determine the time of ovulation. The vaginal mucosa can be examined using a flexible endoscope, a pediatric sigmoidoscope, or, in very small dogs, an otoscope. Rigid endoscopes (cystoscopes) are also available for this purpose and for the observation of transcervical insemination. Observation of the vaginal mucosa to determine ovulation timing is referred to as evaluation of vaginal mucosal crenulation.

The increase in estrogen during proestrus leads to vaginal mucosal edema. The mucosa appears swollen and smooth and makes visualization of the vaginal lumen difficult. As the estrogen levels decrease, so does the edema. This decrease in swelling leads to a wrinkling of the vaginal mucosa, called *crenulation*. Initial crenulation indicates the beginning of the LH peak as the estrogen levels drop. After ovulation, marked wrinkling is seen and the vaginal lumen appears open. The disadvantages of determining vaginal mucosal crenulation are the requirements of prior experience, additional equipment, and sedation.

7.4 HORMONAL ASSAYS

7.4.1 Progesterone Assays

Measurement of serum progesterone during the estrous cycle can also be used to determine ovulation. The use of serum progesterone levels to determine ovulation is based on a normal physiologic increase in progesterone from basal concentration levels (<1 ng/dl) to >2 ng/dl just before ovulation. At the time of ovulation, progesterone levels increase to >4 ng/dl; after ovulation, they are even higher (levels vary with number of follicles). Progesterone is secreted by the corpora lutea after ovulation and signals that the follicle has ruptured and released the egg (ovulation has occurred).

Progesterone levels are measured using a serum sample. The commercial laboratory usually performs a radioimmunoassay or chemiluminescence test to determine serum progesterone levels. It is important that the commercial laboratory measure canine progesterone levels because the assay is species specific. This testing is readily available to the practicing veterinarian; however, a disadvantage may be the turnaround time for obtaining results. Obtaining results over holidays and weekends also may be problematic. Choosing a laboratory that performs the assay daily, allows overnight delivery of samples, and is willing to phone, fax, or email results daily is recommended. Planning is important to ensure that the laboratory will be available when needed. Laboratories that perform this service may be readily found locally or online. Some offer chilled semen service along with progesterone assays.

In-house tests that measure canine progesterone are available. Most require a serum or plasma sample. All require refrigeration and have a shelf life of about 60 to 90 days. The manufacturer's directions must be followed carefully for each test. Samples must be prepared properly because hemolysis may cause a false reading in some tests. Lipemia may also cause false readings on some tests; before these tests are used, the animal may need to be fasted. The tests usually come with standard positive and negative samples for comparison. Results are given as a range rather than a specific number value. The available tests are the PreMate (Camelot Farms, College Station, TX), K9-Proges-Check (Endocrine Technologies, Newark, CA), Status Pro (Synbiotics, San Diego), and Target Canine Ovulation Testing Kit (BioMetallics, Princeton, NJ).

7.4.2 Luteinizing Hormone Assays

The accuracy of determining ovulation timing can be improved by adding an in-house LH assay to the progesterone assay. The LH assay measures the peak LH level that occurs before ovulation. Canine LH assays are available at some reference laboratories but are expensive and not widely used clinically. However, two in-house assays — the K-9 Ovicheck (Endocrine Technologies) and the Status-LH (Synbiotics) — are available. The K-9 Ovicheck assay is a quantitative assay marketed for research professionals to monitor physiologic and pathologic conditions related to circulating LH. The in-house use of this test is limited by its availability and complexity (it requires a two-step incubation process) and the time needed to complete the assay (3 hours). The Status-LH assay is a semiquantitative ELISA that is more readily available and less time consuming. However, because this test is semiquantitative, the results are either positive or negative. The results turn from negative to positive with an increase in serum LH levels consistent with the LH surge. Daily testing with this kit is required, and because preovulatory peaks can occur, an in-house progesterone assay should also be used to ensure that the LH peak is associated with ovulation. Therefore, the major disadvantage of this assay is that it requires serial serum sampling and must be combined with the progesterone assay for accuracy. Ovulation occurs 2 to 3 days after the LH peak; at this point, the progesterone assay should be >4 ng/dl.

7.4.3 Semen Preparation

Fresh, chilled, or frozen semen may be used for artificial insemination. Semen is collected from male dogs using an artificial vagina and manual stimulation. Latex products should be avoided because latex has been reported to decrease sperm motility.[7] Collected sperm should be analyzed for numbers, viability, motility, and morphology.[4,5] The conception rate is best with fresh semen (80%), followed by chilled (60%) and frozen (50% to 60%), but may vary according to the insemination technique used and the skill of the operator. The conception rate also depends on the proper handling of the semen and the fertility of the bitch.

7.4.4 Semen Analysis

Semen analysis, consisting of a sperm count to determine sperm concentration, motility analysis to determine sperm viability, and morphology analysis to identify sperm abnormalities, is performed to determine semen quality. Sperm concentration varies; therefore, sperm counts are conducted using a 1/100 Unopette dilutor (Becton Dickinson) and a hemocytometer. The diluted semen sample is used to charge the hemocytometer, which is placed under the microscope. The sperm present in the middle square of the nine large squares of the hemocytometer are counted and the number multiplied by 1 million to give the number of sperm cells per milliliter. This is multiplied by the volume of the ejaculate to determine the total number of sperm per ejaculation. Sperm counts of >200 million are usually seen in the rested stud dog. Counts of at least 200 million motile sperm are required for reliable vaginal artificial insemination.

Viability is determined by the amount of sperm with forward motility. Therefore, motility is considered the most important parameter in measuring semen quality. Motility can be analyzed by placing a drop of undiluted semen on a slide and placing it under the microscope for examination at 200 to 400x magnification. At least 70% of the sperm should exhibit forward motility.

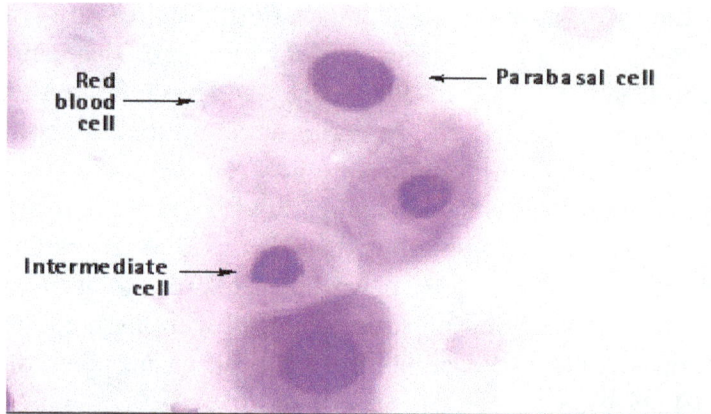

Fig.1: Photomicrographic view (100× magnification) of a vaginal smear taken form a bitch in proestus. Th prabasal cells are small cells with a small nucleus cytioplasm ratio (larger nuclei the largeninte mediate cells have a larger nucleus: cytoplasm ration (smallernuclei) Red blood cells are also seen)

Sperm morphology is analyzed to determine the percentage of morphologically normal sperm in the semen. Abnormal morphologic changes are divided into primary and secondary abnormalities. Primary abnormalities occur in the testes during spermatogenesis. Examples of primary abnormalities are abnormal heads; double midpieces and/or tails; frayed, thickened, bent, kinked or ruptured midpieces; and coiled tails. Secondary abnormalities occur during transit through the epididymis, semen collection process, or preparation of the slide for evaluation. Examples of secondary abnormalities are detached normal heads, detached acrosomes, and bent tails.

Sperm morphology is evaluated by mixing a drop of semen with a drop of eosin-nigrosin stain. The mixture is carefully drawn slowly across the slide like a blood smear and allowed to air dry. Sperm morphology is observed at 1,000x magnification under oil immersion. Normal morphology should be >60% normal sperm that do not present with head, proximal droplet, or tail abnormalities. Primary and secondary defects should constitute <10% and <20%, respectively, of abnormalities seen. Morphologic abnormalities in more than 20% of sperm have been reported to lead to a decrease in litter size.

7.4.4.1 Fresh Semen

Fresh semen has a short life span without preservatives and an energy source. Fresh semen can be immediately instilled by artificial insemination methods if the female has already undergone ovulation timing.

7.4.4.2 Chilled Semen

Frozen or chilled semen can be used if the male dog is not at the same location as the bitch. To prepare chilled semen, fresh semen is centrifuged to make a pellet, which is resuspended in a commercial extender that serves as an energy source for the spermatozoa. The semen is slowly chilled for an hour to preserve the longevity of the sperm during transport. The method used for further preparation and packaging depends on the semen supplier. Chilled semen must be shipped overnight or as soon as possible (ideally in 24 hours) to the owner of the female dog that is to be bred. Testing to determine ovulation timing must be conducted before the semen is shipped.

7.4.4.3 Frozen Semen

Frozen semen is initially prepared in the same way as chilled semen. The extender for frozen semen contains glycerol to prevent damage to the sperm during the freezing procedure. After the semen has been chilled for an hour, it is placed in straws or pelleted and frozen using dry ice or liquid nitrogen, depending on the semen supplier. The frozen semen samples must be labeled with the stud dog's name or other identification and the date of freezing. Semen prepared in this manner can be shipped frozen for use at a later date; therefore, ovulation timing is not necessarily performed before the semen is shipped. Frozen semen must be kept at -4°F (-20°C) until needed and must be used immediately after being thawed. The sperm have decreased viability after the freezing process and must be placed directly into the uterus. Therefore, frozen semen cannot be used with intravaginal insemination.

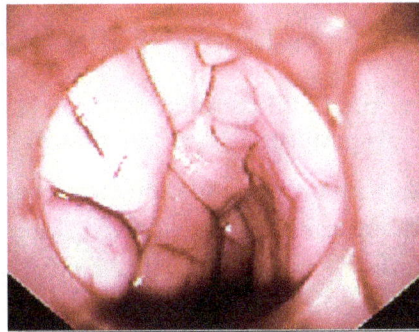

Fig. 2: Endoscopic view of baginal mucosal folds before ovulation the progesterone level is just beginning tot rese (1.3 ng/dl)

Frozen and chilled semen should be prepared by an American Kennel Club (AKC)-recognized collection and storage facility for registration of the litter.[8] There are 160 AKC-recognized collection and storage facilities in the United States. The names and locations of these facilities are available on the AKC Web site. It is important that the owner of the female dog to be bred keep in close contact with the semen supplier and veterinarian to coordinate artificial insemination at the most fertile time of estrus.

7.5 METHODS OF ARTIFICIAL INSEMINATION

Two methods of artificial insemination are described in the literature: intravaginal and intrauterine. The intravaginal method involves instillation of semen into the vagina using a syringe and a long plastic (insemination) catheter. Insemination catheters for species other than dogs (e.g., goats, cows, horses) may be used. The catheter is introduced into the vulva and advanced as far as possible into the vagina. When the catheter cannot be advanced any further, a syringe containing the semen is attached. The bitch is held at a 45° angle with her hind feet in the air while the semen is injected. The syringe is removed, and the bitch remains with her hind end elevated for 15 to 20 minutes to allow gravity to assist sperm transportation to the uterus. A gloved finger may be inserted into the vagina to gently stroke (feather) the vaginal walls to try to stimulate vaginal contractions to assist in moving the sperm cranially toward the cervix. This procedure requires little experience and can be used for multiple serial inseminations daily or every other day. The main disadvantage is that frozen semen cannot be used for this procedure.

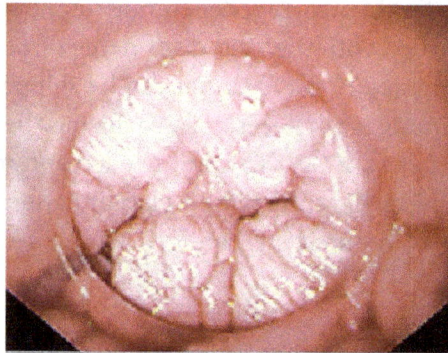

Fig.4: Endoscopic vies of vaginal fold crenulations seen at ovulation. The neasured progesterone level was 4 ng/dl

Transcervical insemination involves instillation of semen into the uterus through the cervix. There are two methods described for transcervical insemination. The Scandinavian or Norwegian approach requires the use of a specialized metal catheter with a nylon sheath. The special catheter and sheath are introduced through the vulva into the cervix, which has been located by abdominal palpation. When the operator is sure that the catheter and sheath are in the cervix, the sheath is removed. The other transcervical method, known as the New Zealand approach, involves mild sedation and a rigid endoscope (cystocope) with a special port that allows visualization of the cervix and placement of an 8-Fr polypropylene catheter into the cervix. Using either transcervical technique, the semen is injected via syringe into the uterus after placement of the catheter. The bitch is then handled similarly to the intravaginal approach. The advantage of the transcervical approach is that because the semen is placed into the uterus, fresh, chilled, or frozen semen can be used. It is also safe enough to be used daily or every other day because only mild sedation may be required. The main disadvantage of transcervical insemination is that both procedures require skill and special equipment.

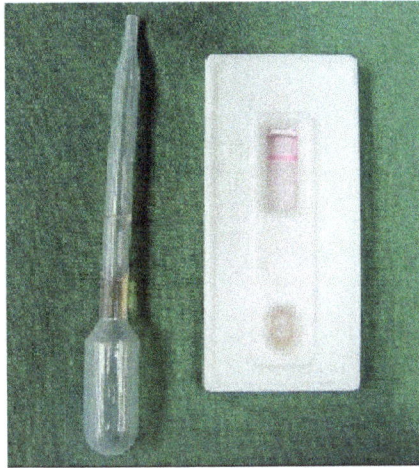

Fig. 5: Results of a negative LH assay using a membrane – based LH test kit.

Surgical intrauterine instillation of semen involves direct injection into the uterus by surgical laparotomy. This procedure requires general anesthesia, a small abdominal incision to exteriorize the uterus, and incision into the uterus to instill the fresh, chilled, or frozen semen. Its major advantage is that it allows the operator to directly observe the injection of the semen into the uterus. However, it requires anesthesia and surgery. Therefore, it is usually only performed once because repeated surgical procedures and anesthesia place the bitch and puppies at risk. Furthermore, this procedure may be banned in some countries as inhumane.

7.6 ROLE OF THE TECHNICIAN

As an assistant to the veterinarian, the technician needs to know what tests may be conducted and which insemination procedure will be used as well as the supplies and equipment needed for each. In some cases, the technician is involved with the prebreeding or breeding soundness examination. The technician may also have the responsibility of preparing and possibly reading slides for vaginal cytology, collecting samples and conducting in-house LH and progesterone assays, or collecting and mailing samples for commercial laboratory assays for progesterone and receiving the results. The technician may also be responsible for keeping up-to-date on what laboratory tests are available and which are preferred based on previous clinic experience.

8

DAIRY GENETIC IMPROVEMENT AND ARTIFICIAL INSEMINATION

8.1 ARTIFICIAL INSEMINATION AND DAIRY CATTLE

⦿ The use of artificial insemination (AI) in dairy cattle is common practise in most countries around the world. AI was introduced during the 1940s following a variety of research trials that were initiated following the birth of the first calf resulting from artificial insemination in Canada in February 1936. Following a relatively slow period of producer acceptance, the use of AI in dairy cattle escalated starting in the late 1960s to a peak in the 1980s after which time it has tended to plateau. Accurate statistics regarding the use of AI are difficult to obtain since a portion of the inseminations are performed by AI technicians while others are performed by herd owners themselves using purchased semen. In general terms, however, the total percentage of dairy cattle in Canada bred artificially reached the 50% mark only in 1975, but from there it quickly grew to approximately 75% during the subsequent decade, where it is estimated that it remains today on an entire population basis. In addition to the increasing acceptance of AI by dairy producers as the preferred method for breeding their heifers and milking cows, other related advancements also were important. These include the improvements in semen processing procedures, especially the use of frozen semen and semen straws, as well as the introduction of young sire testing programs by AI companies .

⦿ Herdbook registered animals serve as the foundation for breed improvement programs and among all animals registered in the dairy cattle breed association herdbooks the percentage that are progeny of AI sires first reached the 90% level in 1987 (Fig. 1). In addition to Herdbook registration to record the identity and ancestry of each animal in the breed, two other data-recording programs have been critical to successful breed improvement over the years, namely milk recording and type classification. Currently, approximately 63% of all dairy cows in Canada are enrolled on a milk recording program, which basically involves the recording of milk production, fat and protein percentages and somatic cell counts for each milking cow in the herd on a monthly basis as well as production-related events such as dates of calving, drying off, culling, etc. For type classification, each breed association offers a program whereby a professional classifier visits the herd and appraises the physical conformation characteristics of each cow in first lactation for a list of approximately 30 traits. At the request of the herd owner, older cows may be re-evaluated and can receive an official reclassification.

◉ The Canadian Dairy Network (CDN) was established in 1995 as the national genetic evaluation centre for dairy cattle in Canada and as such maintains a national database consisting of insemination, herdbook registration, milk recording and type classification data for the Ayrshire, Brown Swiss, Canadienne, Guernsey, Holstein, Jersey and Milking Shorthorn dairy breeds. As an indication of the relative population size of each breed, 92.71% of the herdbook registrations during 2000 were Holsteins while the other percentages were 3.43% Ayrshire, 2.82% Jersey and a combined total of about 1% for the other four breeds. On a quarterly basis, CDN calculates and releases genetic evaluations of bulls and cows for each dairy breed based on sophisticated genetic evaluation systems that evolve over time as research results and new methodologies become available. The use of such genetic evaluations for purposes of selection and mating impacts the rates of genetic progress achieved in the population.

8.2 REALIZED RATES OF PROGRESS

◉ Rates of phenotypic and genetic progress for dairy cattle in Canada have been significant and steadily increasing. While the number of dairy farms in Canada decreased from over 120 000 in 1971 to only 20 000 today, 30 yr later, Fig. 2 shows that the average lactation milk yield per cow has increased by 69% over the same time period (CDN 2002). For cows born since 1980, when most were also recorded for protein yield, the average rate of phenotypic progress per year in Holsteins has been 200 kg milk, 7.0 kg fat and 6.3 kg protein, expressed on a mature equivalent (ME) basis. More recently, however, the milk components have steadily decreased from 3.74% fat and 3.25% protein for cows born in 1989 to 3.63% fat and 3.16% protein 10 yr later.

◉ From a genetic perspective, the average annual rate of progress in the Holstein breed over the past 5 yr has reached 169 kg milk, 5.0 kg fat and 5.3 kg protein, expressed on a ME basis, in conjunction with positive gains for Conformation and other type traits as well . Figure 3 shows the relative rate of genetic progress achieved for various traits in the Holstein cow population, expressed in standard deviation units to allow for comparison across traits, which include production traits, somatic cell score, some major type traits and the Lifetime Profit Index (LPI). Lifetime Profit Index was introduced in 1991 by Agriculture and Agri-Food Canada, which was responsible for dairy cattle genetic evaluations at that time, as the official national selection index for ranking bulls and cows for a combination of important traits. While the specific calculation of LPI has been refined over the years, it has always placed approximately 60% emphasis on production, mainly protein yield, and 40% on longevity, which is mainly represented by type traits. In August 2001, herd life, somatic cell score, udder depth and milking speed were officially incorporated into the LPI formula for all dairy breeds .

⊙ Artificial insemination has a major impact on rates of genetic progress. Once a genetic evaluation based on progeny performance is available, generally when the AI bull is about 5 yr of age, only those considered to be among the best are returned to active service with semen made widely available. The criteria used by the AI organizations to determine which bulls are returned to active service as well as the criteria used by producers to select the AI sires to be used to breed cows in their herd, ultimately impact rates of genetic progress that are achieved. The values in Fig. 3 suggest that protein yield has been the single most important trait considered by producers, based on females born from 1993 to 1998. Partly due to the high genetic correlations amongst milk, fat and protein yields, significant rates of progress have been achieved for all three traits, equalling 0.25, 0.20 and 0.26 standard units per year, respectively. Genetic progress for fat and protein percentage has been negative, however, since there has been little direct selection in favour of high components or against high milk volume. In terms of the type traits, conformation and mammary system have realized gains of 0.15 standard units per year, which closely reflect the breed goal of a relative emphasis on production of 1.5 times that on type, as reflected by the 60:40 ratio in the LPI formula. Relative emphasis on feet and legs and body capacity has been moderately positive but genetic evaluations for somatic cell score have not been available long enough to have resulted in any real genetic progress from direct selection.

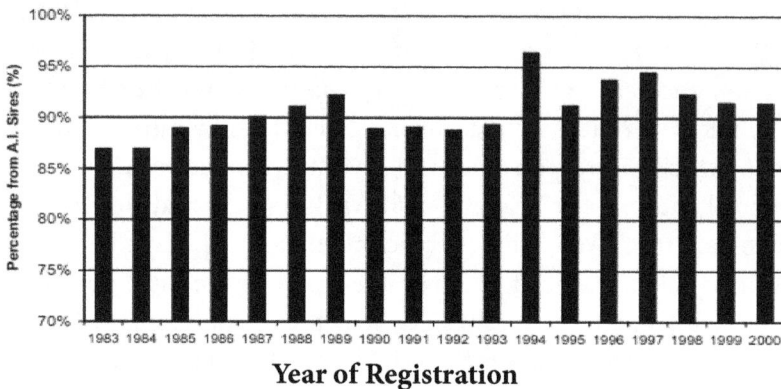

Year of Registration

Fig. 1: The evolution in the percentage of dairy cattle registrations in Canada from artificial insemination sires. Source: Dairy Animal Improvement Statistics published by Agriculture and Agri-Food Canada in 1995 and 2001 (modified to exclude dairy goats).

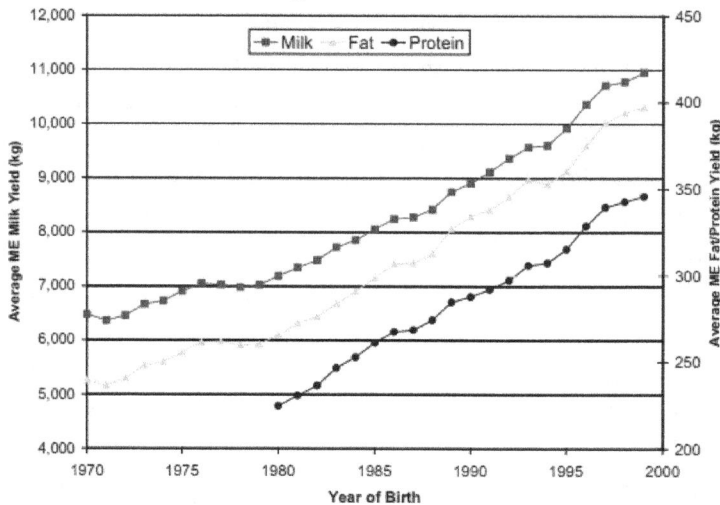

Fig. 2: Trend in the average yield of milk, fat and protein for Holstein cows in Canada, expressed in terms of mature equivalents in kilograms. Averages for protein yield are not shown for cows born prior to 1980 due to incompleteness of data available. Source: Canadian Dairy Network web site (www.cdn.ca) 2002.

- Also, since correlations calculated at the CDN between published bull proofs for somatic cell score and other traits are below 20% for all production and type traits with the only exception being udder depth at 27%, genetic gains for somatic cell score through indirect selection for other traits would be slow. With a realized relative selection intensity of 0.28 standard deviation units for LPI, it is obvious that this overall selection index value, in conjunction with protein yield as its primary component, has been the principal tool used by the industry. The fact that AI allows for each bull to have several dozen, or even several hundreds or thousands of daughters distributed in many different herds, is critical to the calculation of accurate genetic evaluations for a wide variety of economically important traits and hence the rapid rates of genetic improvement.

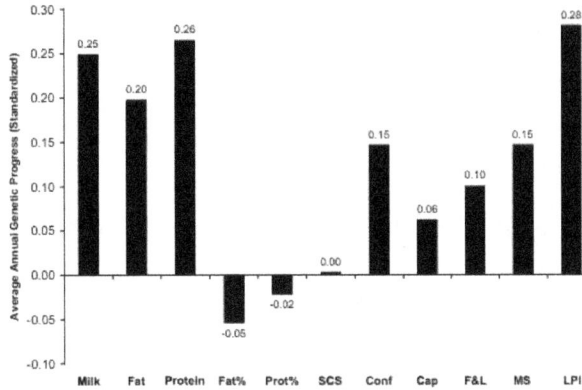

Fig. 3. Average annual genetic progress achieved in the most recent 5-yr period (i.e., cows born from 1993 to 1998), expressed in standard units. Trait abbreviations include Milk = Milk Yield, Fat = Fat Yield, Protein = Protein Yield, Fat% = Fat Percentage, Prot% = Protein Percentage, SCS = Somatic Cell Score, Conf = Conformation, Cap = Capacity, F&L = Feet and Legs, MS = Mammary System and LPI = Lifetime Profit Index.

8.3 FOUR PATHWAYS OF GENETIC PROGRESS

The rate of annual genetic gain is dependent upon four factors:

- ⦿ The genetic variability in the population for the trait of interest,

- ⦿ The degree of selection intensity that is applied when choosing the parents of each future generation from within the current population,

- ⦿ The level of accuracy associated with information used to identify the genetically superior males and females in the current population, and

- ⦿ The generation interval between the birth of the parents compared to the progeny. Genetic gain is maximized when the genetic variability, selection intensity and accuracy are the highest possible and the generation interval is minimized.

More specifically, there are four distinct pathways for genetic selection including (a) the selection of sires to produce sons (SS), (b) the selection of dams to produce sons (DS), (c) the selection of sires to produce daughters (SD), and (d) the selection of dams to produce daughters (DD). The overall annual rate of genetic gain can be calculated by summing the genetic superiorities associated with each of the four pathways and then dividing by the sum of the generation intervals for the four pathways.

Since AI is a technology that allows bulls to have many more progeny than through natural breeding, the impact of AI on rates of genetic improvement is most obvious through the SS and SD pathways. Indirectly, however, the usage of AI allows for more accurate genetic evaluations of both males and females, therefore increasing the accuracy of genetic selection in the DS pathway as well. Although the same is true for the DD pathway, a very low rate of selection intensity for that pathway results due to the fact that most producers breed all available females in the herd and generally raise all heifers that are born, therefore having a minor contribution to the total rate of genetic gain realized in dairy cattle breeding.

8.3.1 Sires of Sons (SS) Pathway

The selection of sires to produce the next generation of young bulls for AI progeny test programs represents the major pathway for achieving genetic progress. Assuming relatively little change in genetic variance over time within a population, this pathway is very important when accurate genetic evaluations are used by AI personnel to identify only the most elite sires of the breed to use as sires of sons and to produce those sons as quickly as possible to minimize the generation interval.

In terms of genetic evaluations, there is no doubt that significant improvements in the calculation methodologies have taken place and increased the accuracy of the results for bulls and cows. Key examples of methodology improvements include the move from "sire" models (Schaeffer et al. 1975) to "animal" models (Robinson and Chesnais 1988) for production and type traits in 1989, therefore providing genetic evaluations for cows in addition to those for bulls, and then the implementation of the Canadian Test Day Model (Schaeffer et al. 2000) for production traits in February 1999.

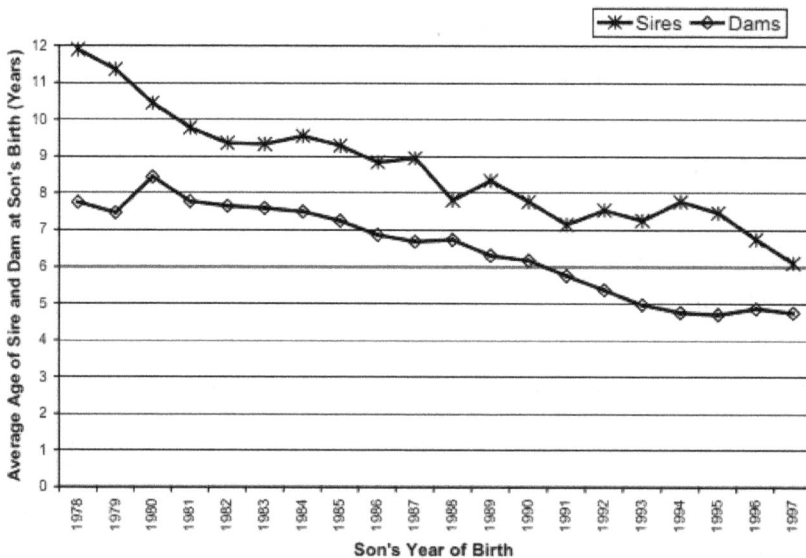

Fig. 4. Trend in the average age of sires and dams at the time of their son's birth for Holstein AI progeny test sires born from 1978 to 1997, reflecting the decrease in generation interval for the sires of sons (SS) and dams of sons (DS) pathways.

The two other components of the SS pathway include the intensity of selection and the generation interval. Although it is difficult to retrospectively evaluate the selection intensity applied over the years without knowing the ranking or relative superiority of each bull in the population when it was selected as a sire of sons, the trend in generation interval for the SS pathway can be examined. Figure 4 shows the average age of the sire at the birth of its sons for young bulls progeny tested in Canada and born between 1978 and 1997. The steady decrease in the average age of the sire at the birth of their son, and therefore the generation interval, has been considerable at an average rate of approximately 3 mo per year, which translates to an average of 3.3% per year. AI young sires born before 1980 were from sires that averaged over 11 yr of age while the interval between the birth of the sire and their AI sons for the most recent years of proven bulls is about 6.5 yr, representing a 40% decrease in the generation interval for the SS pathway.

8.3.2 Dams of Sons (DS) Pathway

Figure 4 also presents the trend in age of the dams at the birth of their sons for bulls that entered AI progeny test programs in Canada. For this DS pathway, the generation interval has also decreased by 40% during the past 20 yr, at an annual rate of about 2.4 mo from approximately 8 yr to less than 5 yr. Obviously, the current availability of relatively accurate genetic evaluations for bulls and cows gives greater confidence to AI personnel who select the young sires. As a result, they are generally using sires immediately when they are first proven combined with first and second lactation cows to produce the next generation of progeny test sires.

8.3.3 Sires of Daughters (SD) Pathway

The sire selection decisions made by producers for breeding the heifers and cows in their herd ultimately has a major impact on the genetic make-up of the cow population and the rate of genetic progress achieved. The generation interval for the SD pathway, as presented in Fig. 5, has also been significantly decreasing during the past decades. The average age of the sire at the birth of their daughters was 7.5 yr for Holstein cows born near 1980, but this has decreased to approximately 6 yr for heifers born in the most recent years.

In Canada, the number of Holstein young sires progeny tested annually has more than doubled in 20 yr from approximately 200 for bulls born in the early 1980s to over 400 in recent years. Based on the current number of daughters for each sire, a retrospective analysis was done to identify the percentage of each year's group of young sires that were subsequently returned to active AI service. For purposes of this analysis, bulls that have less than 200 daughters were considered as not having been widely used following receipt of their progeny test proof at approximately 5 yr of age. Figure 6 shows how the percentage of proven AI Holstein bulls that were returned to active service has changed over the years for bulls first proven since 1985. While there seems to be some year-to-year variation, presumably due to a group of newly proven sons from an elite sire such as the sons of Hanoverhill Starbuck proven in 1990 and 1991 or the sons of Madawaska Aerostar proven in 1996, a general trend of increased selection intensity exists. For bulls proven prior to 1988, the average "return to active service" rate was 15.2%, which decreased to 10.5% for bulls proven between 1988 and 1991 and then to less than 5% for bulls proven thereafter. A negative impact of this increased selection intensity is the narrowing of the genetic base within the population as reflected by increased levels of inbreeding. Statistics at the CDN have shown that the average level of inbreeding in Canadian Holsteins has increased from 2.5% in 1990 to nearly 5.0% today, yielding a rate of + 0.25 percentage points per year, compared to an annual rate of increase of approximately + 0.08 percentage points per year for animals born before the 1990s.

As suggested earlier, the genetic superiority and pedigree diversification are important factors that affect the selection intensity applied by AI organizations when determining which proven bulls should be actively promoted and widely offered to producers. Indirectly, the marketing opportunities and the resulting semen sales revenue for each specific AI organization also have an impact. In fact, during 1990, a major marketing agreement was established involving the largest AI organizations in Canada. A key outcome of this agreement was that various AI organizations started to offer semen from superior proven sires even if they did not own the bull, hence the significant reduction in the overall percentage of AI proven bulls proven after 1991 that were returned to active service.

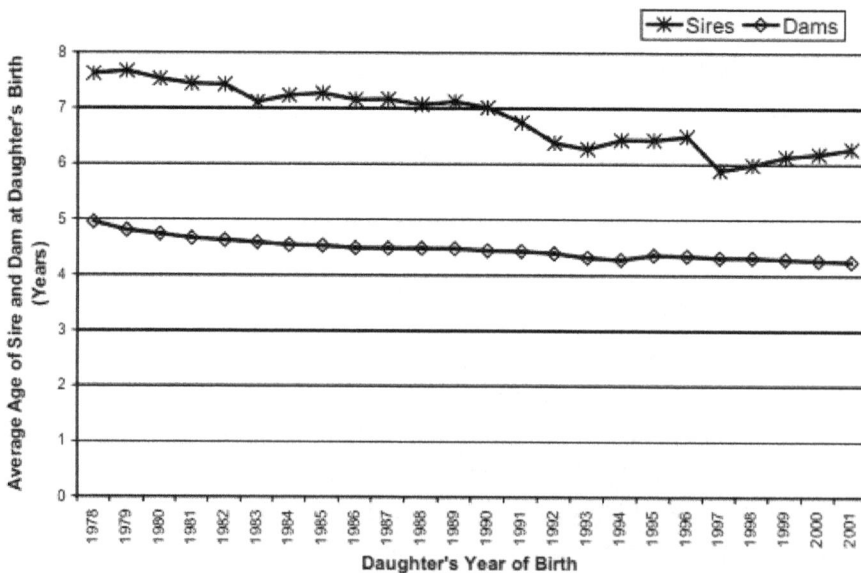

Fig. 5. Trend in the average age of sires and dams at the time of their daughter's birth for Holstein females born from 1978 to 2001, reflecting the decrease in generation interval for the sires of daughters (DS) and dams of daughters (DD) pathways.

8.3.4 Dams of Daughters (DD) Pathway

The generation interval associated with the DD pathway is also presented in Fig. 5. Over the 20-yr period analyzed, the average age of the dams at the birth of their daughters has decreased only approximately 8 mo with the current average being 51 mo of age. As mentioned earlier, this selection pathway is responsible for a very minor portion of the total genetic gain realized in dairy cattle populations.

8.4 IMPACT OF AI ON THE RATE OF GENETIC PROGRESS

There can be no doubt that the use of AI has had a significant impact on the rate of genetic progress realized in dairy cattle populations. On the other hand, AI alone has relatively limited value in dairy cattle breeding since the accuracy, and to a lesser degree the intensity of selection, on the male side would be very low without the availability of data recording programs and genetic evaluation systems to collect and analyze daughter performance. It is the combination of AI with performance recording and genetic evaluations that is critical for rapid genetic gains. The phenotypic trends for production traits in Fig. 2 support this point since the rate of progress in the Holstein breed was much slower prior to 1980 when AI was widely used but genetic evaluations based on a Best Linear Unbiased Prediction sire model became available in Canada only in 1975.

The combination of AI in conjunction with genetic evaluation of bulls and cows has been the key factor contributing to the important genetic gains realized because one complements the other. The use of AI allows each sire to have several hundreds or thousands of daughters distributed across many herds. Genetic evaluation systems allow the analysis of daughter performance in the different herds for various traits of importance, and identify the genetically superior bulls and cows with a certain level of accuracy. Depending on the level of confidence placed on the resulting genetic evaluations, the selection intensity for choosing parents of the next generation may vary but would be increased compared to not having any genetic evaluations. Nevertheless, the availability of semen from genetically superior sires through AI increases the selection intensity as well as the accuracy of selection. Over time, the increased confidence in the accuracy of genetic evaluations results in the use of younger animals as parents, therefore reducing the generation interval. As highlighted earlier, the generation interval associated with all four pathways of genetic progress has decreased over the past 20 yr by 4.5 yr for SS, 3.25 yr for DS, 1.5 yr for SD and 0.65 yr for DD. According to Rendel and Robertson (1950), the change in the sum of the generation intervals across the four pathways can be used to calculate the resulting change in the annual rate of genetic gain achieved. Taking the generation intervals of 20 yr ago, which summed to 31.5 yr compared to the sum for the current population of 21.6 yr, it can be concluded that annual genetic gain is now 46% higher, based solely on the reduction in generation intervals. Increases in the accuracy and intensity of selection achieved during the past 20 yr due to the combination of AI, performance recording and genetic evaluations are more difficult to quantify through a retrospective analysis of data, but have no doubt been significant as well.

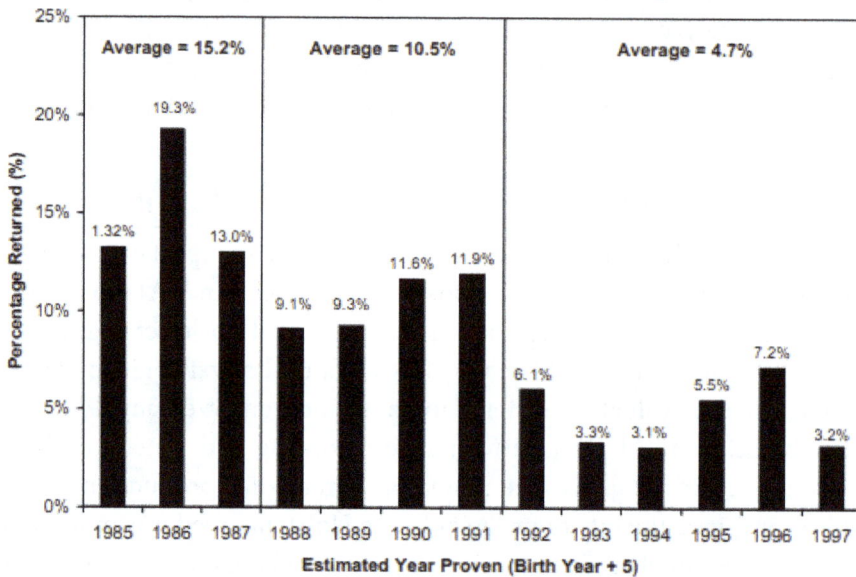

Fig. 6: Percentage of proven AI Holstein bulls returned to active service for bulls with an estimated year of first proof since 1985, based on their birth year plus 5 yr.

8.5 ARTIFICIAL INSEMINATION IN DAIRY CATTLE AT A GLANCE

- ◉ Although AI was introduced in Canada over 60 yr ago, it became the standard practice for a high proportion of dairy producers only in the mid 1970s. At about the same time, in 1975, the first BLUP genetic evaluations were introduced in Canada for production traits. Over the past 20 yr, phenotypic progress for production in the Holstein breed has averaged 200 kg milk, 7.0 kg fat and 6.3 kg protein, in terms of mature equivalent yields. During the same time period, the reduced generation interval for each of the four pathways of genetic progress translates to a rate of annual genetic gain that is now 46% higher without any consideration of the increased accuracy and selection intensity that has also occurred. In terms of relative selection emphasis across traits, the Lifetime Profit Index has received the greatest intensity with 0.28 standard deviation units gain per year over the past 5 yr, followed by protein yield at 0.26 standard deviations per year. The relative gain for protein compared to overall conformation, at 0.15 standard deviations per year, coincides with the general breeding goal of 60% emphasis on production versus 40% on type as a measure of longevity.

- ◉ Genetic evaluation systems have continuously evolved over the years. Their complexity and sophistication grow as the computer processing abilities expand at exponential rates. In addition to data recording and genetic evaluation systems for an increased number of important traits, the enhanced accuracy of resulting evaluations for bulls and cows allows for increasing rates of genetic progress. In the future, AI will continue to be a critical component of the genetic gains possible in dairy cattle breeding but it will be complemented by other reproductive technologies aimed at further reducing generation intervals and increasing the accuracy and selection of intensity, especially on the female side.

9

ADVANCES IN CRYOPRESERVATION OF BULL SPERM

9.1 INTRODUCTION: AN OVERVIEW

There is an urgent need to improve the efficiency and sustainability of producing animals for food in the face of the ever-increasing world population. Increasing the fertility of livestock, especially cattle, around the world is important for overcoming this problem. Improved understanding of mechanisms and challenges of reproductive technologies are vital for improving the viability of the livestock industry. Among such reproductive technologies, Artificial Insemination (AI) is a significant technology that has been utilized to advance livestock farming, allowing for accelerated genetic progress and selection where successful semen

Cryopreservation of semen and artificial insemination have an important, positive impact on cattle production, and product quality. Through the use of cryopreserved semen and artificial insemination, sperm from the best breeding bulls can be used to inseminate thousands of cows around the world. Although cryopreservation of bull sperm has advanced beyond that of other species, there are still major gaps in the knowledge and technology bases. Post-thaw viability of sperm is still low and differs significantly among the breeding bulls.

cryopreservation improves the efficiency and success rate of AI. Sperm cryopreservation procedures are not always efficient because a large number of sperm suffer physiological damage which leads to the loss of fertility following freezing and thawing.

The first reference to sperm cryopreservation dates back to the 1600s. Italian scientist Lazzaro Spallanzani successfully performed artificial insemination on bitches, which resulted in the live birth of three puppies after using cooled sperm in 1784. Another 100 year later in 1899, Russian scientist Ilya Ivanovich Ivanoff developed practical methods of artificial insemination for farm animals. But there was little significant success or any widespread application until a discovery made by Phillips and Lardy in 1940 that poultry egg yolks can protect sperm from cold shock during cooling and maybe added to act as a cryoprotective agent). Salisbury et al. further improved egg yolk usage as an extender by supplementing it with Na-citrate as a buffer to further preserve sperm at low temperature. The next major milestone in the field occurred when Polge et al. uncovered the cryoprotective role of glycerol both at low temperatures and during the freezing process. Other advancements followed in the 1950s with the discovery of different extenders, packaging methods, and procedures which further improved the world-wide use of AI starting in the dairy industry.

Sperm cryopreservation is critical for livestock production because it enables and accelerate the spread of genetic diversity and it facilitates the distribution of genetically superior animals around the world. Due to the importance of cryobiology in reproductive technologies, new protocols are being developed and cryoprotectant agents tested for enhanced cryo-survival of sperm. Progress, however, has not yet reached a desired level because large portions of sperm die during the freezing-thawing processes. During these processes, sperm are faced with physiological and structural challenges due to changes in osmotic balance, oxidative stress, and the formation of intracellular ice crystals, hence, the need for supplements of antioxidants and cryoprotective agents (CPAs). In this paper, the challenges and current techniques to evaluate post-thaw viability of sperm will be discussed as well as the function of CPAs and antioxidants.

9.2 CHALLENGES IN SPERM CRYOPRESERVATION

Cryopreservation of sperm is a sequential process of reduction in temperature, dehydration of the cell, freezing, storage then thawing. Unlike other cells in the body, sperm cells should be less sensitive to their cryopreserving damage due to their low water content and high fluidity of the membranes. Despite this, cryopreservation is detrimental to sperm integrity due to alterations to the membrane structure-function and cell metabolism. Baust et al. summarized the stressors influencing the cells during cooling and freezing stages as following: (1) During cooling, cells are exposed to many harmful effects including metabolic decoupling, ionic imbalance, activation of proteases, cellular acidosis, deprivation of energy, membrane phase transition, destabilization of the cytoskeleton, and production of free radicals or reactive oxygen species (ROS), (2) During process of freezing, sperm are predisposed to detrimental effects of ice crystal formation, hyper-osmolarity, alterations in the cell volume, and protein denaturation (Figure 1).

9.2.1 Membrane Changes

The main cause of cellular injury in cryopreservation is the damage endured by the plasma membrane. Initially, it was assumed that cold shock was associated with the lipid composition of the membrane bilayer). When the temperature is lowered during the cooling process, restrictions of phospholipid lateral movement induce a change from liquid to gel phase causing the membrane to become more rigid and fragile. The phase changes involving the lipid membranes lead to lipid phase separation; thus, proteins are clustered irreversibly.

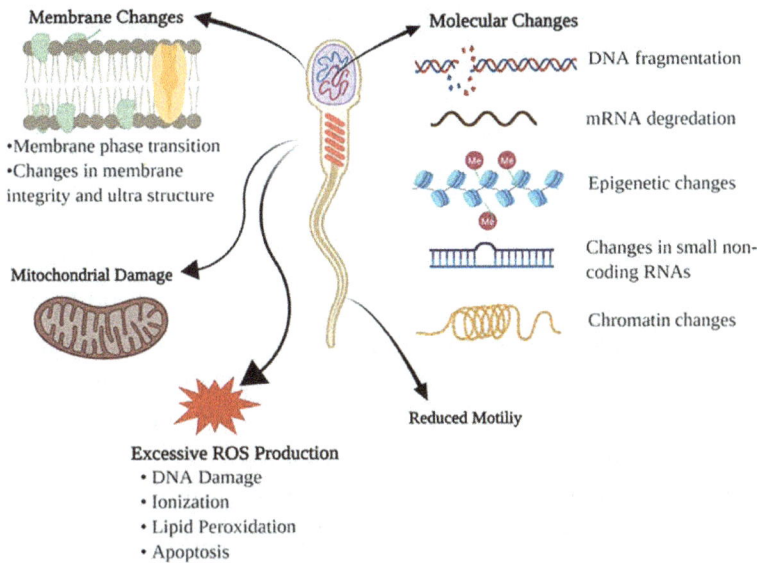

Fig. 1: Detrimental effects of freezing-thawing on a sperm cell. Morphological and physiological effects of freezing and thawing processes on bull sperm are summarized.

9.2.2 Reactive Oxygen Species

During cryopreservation, any changes in mitochondrial membrane fluidity may result in the release of ROS and changes in the membrane potential). Hydrogen peroxide (H_2O_2), nitric oxide (NO), and superoxide anion (O_2-) have positive effects on intracellular signaling, sperm capacitation, and acrosome reactions. Although at the appropriate levels of these molecules play a significant role in sperm physiology, namely capacitation and acrosome reaction, they are detrimental to sperm function at high concentrations due to toxicity. The exact mechanism of ROS generation and function have not been fully characterized in sperm. However, it is known that these molecules are products of incomplete reduction of molecular oxygen, and the toxicity is associated with protein inactivation due to ionization, lipid peroxidation, and DNA damage.

9.2.3 Molecular Challenges

Identification of key molecular determinants of sperm freezability will aid in the development of better extenders and will provide insights to better predict fertility and sperm survival through cryopreservation. Such key determinants of freezability are generally evaluated by changes in parameters such as cell viability, motility and morphology, but current techniques have improved the aspects of novel assessments. Of these indicators of sperm quality, DNA integrity, and chromatin structure have been identified as the crucial factors regarding the ability of sperm to endure the cryopreservation process, and support embryo development. Freezing-thawing adversely affects DNA integrity making the DNA vulnerable and susceptible to molecular and epigenetic modifications, which affect the embryo development. This adverse process has been shown to induce chromatin destabilization which results in DNA fragmentation for boar and avian sperm. DNA damage is likely related to several mechanisms which occur during cryopreservation; double strand breaks due to high levels of ROS production, impairment of DNA repair enzymes, and mechanical stress of genomic regions of the DNA molecule in which chromatin compaction is increased because of cell shrinkage. Apoptosis has been correlated with cryoinjury of sperm DNA and that excessive generation of ROS causes DNA damage. This can be different between fertile and sub-fertile bulls.

Factors including protamine, DNA methylation, and histone modifications take place in an epigenetic state and play critical roles in spermatogenesis. Additionally, the epigenetic factors influence gene expression that is dynamically regulated during cryopreservation. Both mRNA and small non-coding RNA molecules are an important element of intercellular structure and research has shown that they play a role in transcriptional and post-transcriptional regulation of spermatogenesis, while also being involved in reproductive physiology during the freezing-thawing protocols. Sperm RNA quantity can be easily affected during freezing-thawing cycles and some degree of these RNAs remain stable in response to insult. Cryodamage can also cause degradation to mRNAs, and thus disrupt protein function and expression levels of fertility related proteins.

Conventional methods, such as real-time reverse transcription polymerase chain reaction (qRT-PCR) and complementary DNA (cDNA) microarray techniques have been widely used to profile gene products in cryopreserved sperm. However, next-generation sequencing technology has paved the way to the era of transcriptome and the introduction of powerful and rapid new tools for classifying global transcripts of several species. A small number of studies have focused on the global transcriptome of cryopreserved sperm for a few animal species. In the bull, sperm transcripts are present and it was demonstrated that freeze–thaw cycles can lead to changes in transcriptomic profiles between fresh and frozen thawed sperm. Also, cryopreserved sperm show an altered presence of non-coding RNAs including microRNA and piwi-interacting RNA (piRNA). Most recently, it has been shown that non-coding RNAs have been involved in sperm cryoinjuries during cryopreservation and are linked to apoptosis and metabolic activity pathway alterations. Although sperm are transcriptionally silent, the presence of RNA in sperm can provide effects of cryodamage both on sperm and embryo physiology. Recently, cryopreserved sperm has been demonstrated to influence transcriptomic profiles of embryos.

DNA methylation is part of the epigenetic mechanism and refers to the covalent addition of a methyl group to the DNA strand. This mechanism modulates gene expression in a variety of cells. Accurate DNA methylation in sperm is indispensable for early development and embryogenesis. The global level of DNA methylation is correlated with sperm parameters such as motility and concentration while chromatin fragmentation can adversely affect DNA methylation. However, aberrant DNA sperm methylation is linked to infertility in human and bovine. DNA methylation in sperm changes during freezing-thawing cycle that global methylation is increased after cryopreservation. This can also be supported with the regulation of epigenetic related genes which DNA methyl transferase (Dnmt3a and Dnmt3b) genes show *de novo* differential expression levels in cryopreservation. More specifically, a study in zebrafish corroborates that cryopreservation stimulates sperm hypermethylation in the promoters of important genes.

The functional chromatin integrity and packing of sperm genome are critical for the delivery of paternal DNA and epigenetic information to the oocyte. Several mechanical, physiological, and chemical factors can deteriorate chromatin integrity. There is increasing evidence suggesting that the sperm nucleus with altered chromatin structure provides additional information on cryodamage from freezing-thawing which cause alterations including denaturation. These changes influence the fertilizing capability of sperm without affecting functionality parameters. In most species and instances, low quality sperm have partly condensed chromatin which is susceptible to insult by polymerase and nucleases, resulting in DNA damage and is associated with infertility in bull. Methods of freezing and the stage of cryopreservation can influence chromatin structure that it is mostly impaired at the thawing stage of cryopreservation. Also, nuclear sperm alterations are attributed to cycles of freezing and thawing which subsequently link to DNA damage.

9.3 MOLECULAR MARKERS OF SPERM FREEZABILITY

Seminal plasma and sperm proteins play important roles in sperm survival, fertilization, and energy metabolism. Recent studies showed that protein compositions and their expression levels in seminal plasma and sperm are associated with freezability differences among bulls. Some of the bovine seminal plasma proteins bind phospholipids of the sperm plasma membrane and hinder the movement of phospholipids. Expression levels of heat-shock protein (HSP90) were higher in semen with greater cryotolerance, and the levels of the HSP90 in bull sperm were significantly decreased in bull spermatozoa with lower cryotolerance. Holt et al. claim that lower concentrations of heat shock protein A8 (HSPA8) in freezing media cause reduced post-thaw sperm viability, whereas higher concentrations improve plasma membrane integrity.

The cryopreservation process initiates carbonylation of bull sperm proteins. Mostek et al. identified 11 proteins in bull semen (NADH dehydrogenase, ropporin-1, actin-related protein T2, outer dense fiber protein 2, glutathione S-transferase, triosephosphate isomerase, capping protein beta 3 isoform, actin-related protein M1, isocitrate dehydrogenase, cilia- and flagella-associated protein 161, phosphatidylethanolamine-binding protein 4) that they showed significant carbonylation levels during cryopreservation. Jobim et al. found that presence of lipocalin-type prostaglandin D synthase (L-PGDS) is associated with poor freezability of bull sperm. The expression level of an acidic seminal fluid protein (aSFP) is higher in semen from high freezability sperm than that from low freezability. It assumed that aSFP plays a key role in protecting sperm from the damaging effects of oxidative stress by reducing lipid peroxidation.

9.4 EXTENDER DEVELOPMENT

9.4.1 Current State of the Art in Extenders for Bull Sperm

The cold shock endured during freezing and thawing reduces the quality of sperm. The extent of injuries from cold shock vary according to contents of extenders, cryoprotectants used, and species. A number of extenders have been developed to lessen cryodamage and improve post-thaw viability. Extenders based on 20% egg yolk are commonly used to cryopreserve livestock sperm of cattle, buffalo, and pigs. Although egg yolk is known to prevent cell damage during cryopreservation, the presence of substances in yolk granules including high-density lipoproteins (HDL) and minerals inhibit respiration of sperm cells and reduce their motility. However, the low density lipoproteins (LDL) of egg yolk protect sperm from damage by covering the sperm membrane during freezing and thawing. Although most extenders include egg yolk alone, some are supplemented with glycerol, and there are some concerns over biosecurity and the possibility that egg contents might alter sperm structure and physiology.

There have been efforts to develop commercial extenders with defined contents and those that are free of animal products. Recent studies performed by Murphy et al. and Yodmingkwan et al. revealed that plant-based extenders can be efficiently used as alternatives to animal-based extenders in frozen semen to avoid spread of diseases. However, there are conflicting results related to the efficacy of lecithin-based extender for semen freezing. Vidal et al. claimed that there were no significant difference in post-thaw goat semen parameters between semen extended in Soy-lecithin based extender vs. Skim milk-based extender. Aires et al. referred that the Andromed® extender containing soy-lecithin was better when compared to an egg yolk extender in cryopreservation of sperm from Holstein bulls. Additionally, Chelucci et al. reported that soy-lecithin based extender preserves frozen goat semen better than that of an egg yolk based extender. However, according to Muiño et al. a Biladyl® extender containing tris-egg yolk gave better results in terms of survival of sperm that those from Andromed® and Biociphos®. Other researchers claim that Tris-egg yolk-based extender is better in preserving frozen semen than plant-based extenders. Moreover, studies on liposome based extenders have showed its effectiveness over both animal based and plant based extenders in preserving the frozen semen of buffalos (Bubalus bubalis). There is a desperate need for more research and more extensive analyses of sperm as well as follow up studies on pregnancy rates and live births of offspring using sperm cryopreserved with different extenders.

9.4.2 Cryoprotectant Supplementation of Extenders

Nonpenetrating and penetrating cryoprotectants are used to protect sperm cells from physical and chemical stressors caused by ice crystallization. While non-penetrating cryoprotectants such as polymers help with vitrification, penetrating cryoprotectants such as sugars help reduce toxicity. Cryoprotective agents cannot not prevent the changes in membrane phase but they can decrease the rate of dehydration during freezing which then lessen the formation of ice crystals in the cell.

Although glycerol, ethylene glycol, dimethyl sulfoxide, and 1,2-propanediol are all CPA, glycerol is the most commonly used in bovine sperm because it causes dehydration of cells by creating osmotic stimulation. Concentrations of CPAs differ among extenders; skim milk based extenders contain 8%, Tris eggyolk extenders contain 6–7% CPA. Therefore, the volume of intracellular water decreases and the chance of the ice formation reduces. However, glycerol may cause osmotic stress and toxicity. In addition, sugars and polyols are used as cryoprotectants in semen processing. They create hydrogen bonds with membrane lipids; thus, lipids of sperm membrane are stabilized at low temperatures. Milk diluents are commonly used as CPA in bull semen. However, they have the disadvantage of decreasing the visibility of sperm cells under the microscope during sperm evaluation due to fat globules. Cryopreservation procedures cause significant losses of total lipids and phospholipids of sperm cells. Due to the importance of fatty acid composition on membrane fluidity, supplementations of fatty acids to the extender affect freezability. When the egg yolk-based extender was supplemented with docosahexaenoic acid, a major fatty acid in fish oil, sperm post-thaw viability has increased.

More recently, addition of 8% coconut oil as a source of lauric acid to egg yolk based-extender, 5 ng/ml α-linoleic acid to the BioXcell ®, and 20 ng/ml arachidonic acid to tris-citric acid extender enhanced quality of sperm following cryopreservation. Additionally, Iodixanol is commonly used as a medium for density gradient centrifugation. Supplementation of sperm cells with Iodixanol (OptiPrep™) increases motility of buffalo sperm post-thaw. Mechanisms of Iodixanol actions are not clearly understood but it has been assumed that it protects sperm membrane through reducing ice crystal formation.

9.4.3 Antioxidant Supplementation of Extenders

Antioxidants are molecules that inhibit the formation of ROS and lipid peroxidation. Superoxide dismutase, glutathione peroxidase, and catalase are the well-known antioxidants that are significant for sperm function because they protect sperm cells from oxidative stress. Glutathione (GSH) is a powerful antioxidant that protects bull sperm against free oxygen radicals and supplementation of buffalo semen with GSH increased motility, integrity of plasma membrane and cell viability. Another critical antioxidant for sperm integrity is Resveratrol which extinguishes superoxide, hydroxyl, and metal-induced radicals. Therefore, it protects sperm chromatin and membranes from ROS damage. Vitamin E also plays an important role on sperm membrane protection as an antioxidant. Supplementation of semen with vitamin E affects sperm motility, membrane integrity, and membrane potential positively. Endogenous antioxidants present in bovine semen are not sufficient to ensure sperm integrity against oxidative stress in cryopreservation. The supplementation of antioxidants is needed to improve the viability of post-thawed sperm cells. Bovine Serum Albumin (BSA) protects the sperm plasma membrane and acrosome, and physiology such as motility. Sariözkan et al. found that the addition of BSA helped to maintain the cell morphology and acrosome integrity, and increased its catalase (CAT) activity. In addition, methionine is a precursor for glutathione which protects sperm from oxidative damage and is involved in detoxification of the cell. Moreover, the addition of methionine to semen helped to maintain normal sperm morphology. Furthermore, addition of carnitine and inositol to extenders has shown to have a protective influence on acrosome integrity as well as improved sperm motility and reduced DNA damage.

Plant-derived extracts are sources of natural antioxidants with lower cytotoxicity as compared to artificial antioxidants. Khan et al. found that adding green tea extract at an inclusion level of 0.75% protected the plasma membrane and increased motility rates of cryopreserved spermatozoon. The addition of Spirulina maxima Extract (SME), a microalga, to extender has exhibited positive effects on post-thaw semen parameters including sperm motility and morphology, and marked reduction in ROS synthesis. Other natural compounds have been found to act as an antioxidant. Trehalose is a sugar that functions as an antioxidant and wa s shown to protect the structure of the sperm cell from oxidative and cold shock damage. The addition of 100 mM of trehalose into semen extender improved sperm post-thaw motility, integrity of the membrane, and the activities of CAT and GSH. Furthermore, supplementing semen extender with 2 μg/ml of selenium, a potent antioxidant, improved morphology, and integrity of cryopreserved sperm.

9.4.4 Vitamins and Other Supplementations of Extenders

Vitamins, known for their antioxidant properties, along with other compounds may be utilized to combat cryo-damage and improve overall post-thaw quality of sperm. Vitamin C has been tested as an additive to extenders for the purpose of improving sperm quality after the harsh challenges that are brought upon the cells by cryopreservation. Vitamin C acts as an electron donator, to neutralize free radicals that are generated from normal metabolic activity in addition to environmental challenges. This ability to donate electrons allows for the reduction of oxidative stress from ascorbate free radicals (AFR). In a study performed by Mittal et al. supplementation of 5 mm vitamin C to pooled bull ejaculates significantly improved seminal characteristics and significantly decreased the number of observed abnormal sperm as compared to the control group measurements. Vitamin C supplementation to sperm extenders has also been studied in buffalo bulls and has shown greater post-thaw motility and percent of intact plasma. Feeding animals with ascorbic acid has also shown significant increases in physical semen characteristics of ejaculate volume and sperm concentration, contributed to difference in scrotal circumference, reaction time, and testicular volume, while also improving sperm output characteristics such sperm motility, and total counts for Egyptian buffalo bulls.

Herbal extracts and supplements are another up and coming area of untapped potential for the animal reproduction industry. Silymarin is one such extract with potent antioxidant properties that comes from the milk thistle plant Silybum marianum . Little research has been conducted utilizing silymarin in cattle but recently in a study performed by El-Sheshtawy and El-Nattat the supplementation of silymarin improved preservability of sperm in both chilled and frozen bull semen samples. Rosemary, Rosmarinus officinalis, a common household herb, has also been investigated as a potential cryoprotectant. In a study performed by Daghigh-Kia et al., researchers supplemented bull sperm samples with rosemary extract, GSH, and a combination of the two to determine how the semen would be affected after being subjected to cryopreservation procedures. Results showed that the inclusion of the rosemary extract treatment and the combination treatment improved post-thaw characteristics of bull semen. Semen supplements discussed in that section have been summarized in Table 1.

Table 1. Extender development for sperm cryopreservation.

Supplement	Functions/Effects
CRYOPROTECTANTS	
Egg yolk	Low density lipoproteins (LDL) in egg yolk bind cell membrane and form an interfacial film during the freezing process
Milk	Protein fraction of skim milk protects sperm cells from cryo-injury
Glycerol	Responsible for membrane lipid and protein rearrangement
Ethylene glycol	Reduce intracellular ice formation by increasing dehydration at lower temperature
Dimethyl sulfoxide	
Propylene Glycol	
Trehalose	Replace the bound water surrounding macromolecules and protectively hydrate those macromolecules by substituting for water
Polyols	Create hydrogen bonds with membrane lipids; thus, lipids of sperm membrane are stabilized at low temperatures
Fatty acids	
• Docosahexaenoic acid (Fish oil)	Increase post thaw viability, motility, and acrosome integrity by improving plasma membrane fluidity and integrity
• Lauric acid (Coconut oil)	
• a-linoleic acid	
• Palmitic acid	
• Oleic Acid	
Iodixanol	It assumed that protects sperm membrane through reducing ice crystal formation; thus, increases post-thaw sperm motility
Butylated hydroxytoluene	Enhances motility, acrosomal integrity, and membrane integrity by increasing membrane fluidity and reducing activity of the lipid peroxyl radicals

ANTIOXIDANTS	
Glutathione	Glutathione supplementation increase motility, plasma membrane integrity, and viability
Resveratrol	Extinguishes superoxide, hydroxyl, and metal-induced radicals. Therefore, it protects sperm chromatin and membranes from ROS damage
Vitamin E	Affects sperm motility, membrane integrity, and membrane potential positively
Bovine Serum Albumin	Helps to maintain the cell morphology and acrosome integrity, and to increase its catalase (CAD activity
Methionine	Maintain normal sperm morphology
Carnitine Inositol	Improve acrosome integrity, sperm motility, and reduce DNA damage
Spirulina Maxima Extract	Increase the motility and viability of sperm cells, and reduce ROS synthesis and protect DNA structure
Selenium	Improve morphology and integrity of cryopreserved sperm
VITAMINS	
Vitamin C	Vitamin C supplementation increase post-thaw motility and percent of intact plasma

9.5 TECHNIQUES TO EVALUATE SPERM QUALITY

Comprehensive analyses of sperm by using integrated diverse methods are necessary to assess the cell morphology at the molecular and cellular levels that are linked to cell function. For examples, most relevant, advanced, standardized techniques should be applied correctly to capture sperm cell, genetic, functional, and epigenetic content. To improve cryopreservation, accurate predictor of sperm motility, viability, membrane functionality, mitochondrial activity, and apoptosis parameters should be assessed by contemporary techniques.

9.5.1 Microscopy

Light Microscopy has been a commonly used tool to evaluate basic quality parameters of semen including sperm motility, morphology, membrane integrity, and concentration. *Fluorescent microscopy* has been an essential tool in biology and reproductive sciences, because of wide array of fluorochromes. The use of fluorescence labeling enables identification of sub-microscopic cellular components. Fluorescent microscopy has been extensively used to analyze sperm viability, the sperm membrane, acrosome, and chromatin. In this microscopy method, cellular components of sperm function are stained with fluorescent probes to examine the DNA, membranes, or lectins. Sperm viability assay can be analyzed by fluorescence microscopy using LIVE/DEAD commercial kits, which are DNA-binding fluorescent stains (SYBR-14) and membrane-permeant stain (PI), respectively. Acrosome integrity can be analyzed using the sperm acrosome molecular marker *Pisum sativum* agglutinin linked to fluorescein isothiocyanate (FITC-PSA). Terminal transferase dUTP nick-end-labeling (TUNEL) can also be used to evaluate apoptosis by flow cytometry and fluorescence microscopy.

Laser Confocal fluorescence microscopy is a technique that obtains three-dimensional (3D) optical resolution with depth of focus and provides protein distributions in cellular compartments. The advantages of confocal microscopy are that it recognizes fluorescence in individual cells, provides multispectral flexibility, and avoids out-of-focus suppression. In a confocal fluorescent microscope, excitation of the specimen beam by a laser is concentrated through the first pinhole aperture and then the emitted light is obtained and focused by the second pinhole and subsequently measured by a detector. Depending on the instrument type, confocal setup is required before each experiment; excitation laser is set considering maximal excitation and emission of each fluorochrome. To focus on sperm, the objective is set depending on sperm size, and parameters such as pinhole and gain voltage are adjusted for fluorochrome tested. For the acquisition of images of sperm, instrument acquisition parameters such as bit dept, thickness, and image format are adjusted for detection. Confocal microscopy is used to evaluate sperm characteristics such as the acrosome, chromatin, and membrane. More specifically, cytoskeletal proteins, such as, spectrin, tubulin and actin in the head of sperm can be examined by laser confocal fluorescence microscopy, likewise, expression of surface proteins in sperm cells can be evaluated. This microscopy allows observation of sperm movement, but lack of qualification and quantification of various characteristics, and provides accurate visualization of mitochondria; can be used to analyze mitochondria functionality at the single-cell level, while also can be adjusted for tracking of motion of sperms with active mitochondria. In addition, it can be applied to ascertain localization of lipid peroxidation and ROS in sperm.

Electron Microscopy (EM) uses the electron as a tool to utilizes a beam of accelerated electrons to develop a specimen image. This technique provides higher magnification and resolution than light microscopy. In light microscopy, visible light is used to magnify the image of a specimen by using optical lenses that are the range of 10–1,000 times magnification. EM is performed in a vacuum and directly focuses an electron beam on the subject and images are magnified by the means of electromagnetic lenses. This microscopy technique has the advantage of using shorter wavelength of electrons at accelerating voltage. EM considerably expands our understanding of ultrastructure and morphological characteristics of sperm. The two most common electron microscopes are Transmission electron (TEM) and scanning electron (SEM). In these advanced microscopes, electromagnetic lenses are used to focus the electron beam on the image. Essentially, TEM sends off electrons via ultrathin sample to detector and generates two-dimensional image, while SEM scans the secondary electrons reflected from the specimen's surface and composition to create a three-dimensional image. SEM is used to examine the surface of sperm cell at low resolution with extensive magnification. SEM is advantageous when investigating adverse effects of cryopreservation on sperm morphological changes. TEM can be applicable to reproductive medicine and the investigation of structure and function of sperm. EM has beneficial uses in the diagnosis of sperm morphological defects.

Holographic microscopy and Raman spectroscopy have a holographic microscopy format where samples are visualized by laser light, and the obtained images are used to define the position, orientation, and the 3D structures of a microscopic sample. This technique provides label-free, no contact visualization, and high-resolution recording with numerical focusing which allows for 3D quantitative imaging of specimen and enables live cell applications on sperm morphology and motility. Holographic microscopy can be employed to evaluate morphology and integrity of bull sperm. Recently, computational, lens-free, and on-chip microscopy tools have been developed to track sperm heads and trajectories in second ranges for each frame Human sperm structure can also be assessed by holographic microscopy. Recently, this high-throughput technique with developed image reconstruction was used to track sperm heads and tail in 3D locomotion. Raman spectroscopy is a useful technique that facilitates the study of biochemical changes of cellular components. The Raman spectroscopy technique is sensitive and non-destructive and relies on direct inelastic light scattering from a laser source in which frequency of photons is directed on a sample and scattered photon is detected as Raman effect. This frequency provides detailed information about identificated molecules from vibrational transitions with molecular interaction and composition, such as proteins and DNA in normal and abnormal human sperm. Raman microspectroscopy has the capability of evaluation of chemical changes and molecular features of human and bovine sperm cells. Additionally, it offers an analysis of live sperm with physiological status. Raman spectroscopy can be combined with holographic microscopy to assess sperm quality with relation to morphological and biochemical properties.

9.5.2 Computer-Assisted Sperm Analysis (CASA)

The CASA system, first established in 1980, has evolved into an accurate computer-based technique and software which provides quantitative measurements to assess the sperm motility and kinematics objectively and precisely. This technique uses the principle of capturing continuous images of motile sperm from a microscopic field and converts images into video images with different acquisition rates (frames s-1, Hz). Captured images are scanned to be visualized through dark field or negative-high-phase contrast in order to track motion of each individual sperm considering intensity of frame in pixels and the head. CASA provides motility parameters [progressive motility (%), total motility (%)] and kinematic characteristics for evaluation of sperm such as velocity, linearity, and lateral displacement which defines trajectory. This widely used measure of sperm movement includes velocities such as straight-line (VSL), curvilinear (VCL), average pathway (VAP), linearity of forward progression (LIN, ratio of VSL to VCL), and Amplitude of lateral head displacement (ALH). With high quality hardware and open-source software, current CASA systems are also more useful for the measurement of sperm morphometry (dimension) while also allowing for assessment of sperm viability, concentration, morphology, and degrees of DNA fragmentation.

9.5.3 Flow Cytometry

Flow cytometry (FC) is an outstanding system which has made it possible to analyze thousands of single cells in a short time. Flow cytometry permits analyses of large numbers of sperm cells as well as individual cells with physical characteristics of a single spermatozoon measured by a fluorescent compound. It is composed of fluidics, optics, and electronics systems, which uses the measurement of physical optics and chemical fluorescence characteristics of particles in a fluid when it is passes through a laser source.

In brief, this technique requires a small amount of sperm cell suspension and particle samples labeled with fluorescent markers in suspension which can be injected into a flow cell in the instrument. Subsequently, the fluorescence is absorbed and wavelengths of fluorescence from particle emission are detected by two optic lenses, generating measurement of fluorescent bands. During data collection, non-sperm scatter is gated out, considering characteristics of spermatozoon and fluorescence is subtracted from the total fluorescent intensity. Two types of flow cytometry systems are available, one of which having sorting capabilities (fluorescence activated flow cytometry-FACS) allows physically separation and purification of cells. The other is non-sorting, which measures fluorescent emission in a highly repeatable, accurate, and sensitive manner. It generates high-throughput data on subpopulations while also capturing the measurements of heterogenous populations such as sperm. The structure of multiple organelles of sperm can be simultaneously evaluated using flow cytometry:

Cell viability analysis helps identify viable and non-viable sperm which are associated with the molecular anatomy and physiology of the membranes. More specifically, during the cryopreservation process, changes in temperature and osmotic stress impair sperm viability because of injury to the plasma membrane. This method uses probes such as ethidium homodimer (EH)), propidium iodide (PI), Yo-Pro-1, and bizbenzimidazole Hoechst 33258 dyes, alone, or in combination with other dyes, to excite lasers. Propidium iodide (PI) is excited with the 488-nm laser and able to penetrate the non-viable sperm through broken plasmalemma, then emit red fluorescence upon binding to nucleic acids. SYBR-14, viability probe, emits green fluorescence from nuclei upon entering active cells, and can be combined with PI. This staining technique can be modified with other stain combinations to assess acrosomal integrity or mitochondrial function. SYBR14-PI staining has been employed to evaluate the effects of cryopreservation on sperm viability in many species, such as bee, stallion, bovine, and fish. Yo-Pro-1 is a green cyanine probe which reaches emission at 509 nm and can be applied to study membrane permeability.

Yo-Pro-1 is combined with a membrane permeable dye ethidium homodimer and carboxyseminaphthorhodal fluor-1 (SNARF-1) to assess membrane stability in cryopreserved sperm. Also, a combination of Yo-Pro-1 and PI can be better practiced than SYBR-14/PI to detect early phase damages in the membrane. Fluorescent probe Hoechst 33258 requires the ultraviolet laser to excite at 352 nm and emits blue fluorescence at 461 nm when bound to the nucleic acid. Hoechst 33258 can be used to determine viable and non-viable sperm and it also provides an option to be combined with other probes leaving the green-red detection available. Hoechst 33342 (H-42) is another cell-permeant nuclear dye that is excited by an ultraviolet laser at 350 nm and emits blue fluorescence at 461 nm after binding to DNA. Recently, this dye has been used with ethidium homodimer to differentiate live and dead sperm cells.

Lately, fixable viability dyes relying on reaction of fluorescence with cytoplasmic amines have become available to detect live and dead cells and applicable for multicolor experiments. Fixable dyes cannot pass through an intact live cell membrane, resulting in a weak staining. However, they can stain amines in the cytoplasm of damaged cells. Zombie Green™, a fixable dye, is excited at 488 nm with a blue laser has a maximum emission at 515 nm. This dye has been tested for evaluation of sperm viability and mitochondrial membrane potential (MMP).

Acrosome integrity, an indication of intactness, is essential for fertilization and the subsequent penetration of sperm into the zona pellucida. Acrosome integrity assays have been widely analyzed by a number of methods such as phase contrast, fluorescence with probes, and electron microscopy. Instead, flow cytometry requires labeled acrosome with lectin probes conjugated with fluorochrome fluorescent isothiocyanate (FITC). For this purpose, due to specificity, *Arachis hypogaea* (peanut) agglutinin (PNA) and *Pisum sativum* (pea) agglutinin (PSA) are the most commonly used lectins. In damaged acrosomes, while PSA lectin recognizes α-D- glucosyl and α-D-mannosyl residues in acrosome and stains acrosomal matrix, PNA binds to the outer acrosomal membrane.

PNA label in damaged or reacted spermatozoa emits green fluorescence, but intact acrosomes cannot yield fluorescence. The integrity of plasma membrane as well as the acrosomal integrity are measured at the same time using the combination of FITC-PSA and PI which has been used in dog and cryopreserved bovine sperm. PNA-FITC staining can be more precise in the detection of acrosome than PSA-FITC. Also, combination of FITC-PNA/PI staining is useful for semen quality, allowing for the assessment of viability, and acrosomal integrity with analysis of live/dead and intact/damaged ratio and evaluation of effects of cryopreservation on acrosomal status .

Mitochondrial activity is an indicator of sperm physiology has been analyzed using fluorochromes with flow cytometry to elucidate mitochondrial function in the sperm. The 3,3- Dihexyloxacarbocyanine iodide-484/501nm [DiOC6(3)], green fluorescence dye, has been previously employed to analyze semen. However, this dye tends to stain other organelles, such as Golgi apparatus, when used at higher concentrations and can be non-specific in determining membrane potential. Rhodamine 123 (R123), a green-fluorescent dye that was used to evaluate MMP, has been replaced by improved dyes such as MitoTracker or JC-1 dyes. R123 cannot differentiate high and low MMP because of high mitochondrial respiratory rates and can lose signals out of sperm cells when the MMP is weak. MMP can be analyzed by using commercial dyes such as MitoTracker which works by permeating the cell and accumulating in the mitochondria. When it is bound to mitochondria, mitochondria steadily emit fluorescence even after the cell dies, thus allowing multicolor labeling in sperm. MitoTracker dyes show a broad range of fluorescence (red, green, orange) and accumulate in active mitochondria after spreading across the plasma membrane. Of these, Carbocyanine-based MitoTracker® Probes, such as MitoTracker Green FM and MitoTracker Red FM, act as a marker for live cells dependent on MMP but cannot be retained after fixation. However, Rosamine-based MitoTracker® Probes (MitoTracker Orange CM-H$_2$TMRos, MitoTracker Orange CMTMRos, MitoTracker® Red CMXRos, MitoTrackerR Red CM-H$_2$XRos) are well-retained after aldehyde fixation. The Rosamine family of reduced MitoTracker dyes, MitoTracker Red CM-H$_2$XRos and MitoTracker Orange CM-H$_2$TMRos, do not emit fluorescence until oxidative respiration occurred and can be used for estimation of oxidation status in sperm cells. These probes have been utilized to assess sperm, specifically MitoTracker Deep Red and MitoTracker Green, have been used to determine MMP. The 5,5,6,6-tetrachloro-1,1,3,3-tetraethylbenzimidazolylcarbocyanine iodide (JC-1), another mitochondrial dye, is more specific to MMP, and enables the differentiation between low and high MMP with dual fluorescence shifting from green to orange. In inactive mitochondria, forming monomers emits green fluorescence (525–530 nm wavelength) after being excited with a blue laser at 488 nm when MMP is low. However, inactive mitochondria with high MMP, form J-aggregates reach maximum spectra at 590 nm and emit orange fluorescence once excited with yellow (561 nm) laser. JC-1 has been used to evaluate semen quality, and to show differences in the sperm mitochondrial function.

9.5.4 Oxidative Stress Analysis

Oxidative stress has detrimental effects on sperm by deteriorating fertilizing ability. This is caused by production of ROS including radicals such as hydroxyl radical (OH), superoxide anion (O2) and non-radical hydrogen peroxide (H$_2$O$_2$). During cryopreservation and thawing, sperm cells undergo cold shock which then leads to excessive ROS and lipid peroxidation . ROS and oxidative species can be detected with better accuracy and reproducibility using flow cytometry as compared to other approaches. The 2, 7-dichlorodihydrofluorescein diacetate (H$_2$DCFDA) is commonly used as ROS indicator to measure intercellular H$_2$O$_2$. Nonfluorescent H$_2$DCFDA penetrates into the cell membrane and becomes stable in the intercellular once cleaved by intracellular esterases.

Upon oxidation, it emits green fluorescence at ~517–527 nm by conversion to fluorescent 2,7-dichlorofluorescein (DCF) form). Dihydroethidium (hydroethidine) is a specific ROS indicator probe that can be employed to detect superoxide production. The reduced form is oxidized by superoxide and emits red fluorescence at 610 nm after intercalating into DNA. This probe can be combined with viability markers to better determine ROS generation in live cells and can be applied to study intracellular ROS in sperm. The 5-(and 6) -chloromethyl-20, 70-dichlorohydrofluorescein diacetate (CM-H_2DCFDA), an oxidative stress probe, shows better retention than H_2DCFDA and measures hydrogen peroxide in intact cells. Upon moving into the cell, CM-H_2DCFDA diffuses into the plasma membrane, and acetates are cleaved by cellular esterases and thiol-reactive chloromethyl group to form 20,70-dichlorodihydrofluorescein (H_2DCF). Then, oxidation of H_2DCF into DCF by H_2O_2 emits fluorescent at 525 nm once excited at 495 nm. This probe is also convenient for the assessment of oxidative stress in bull sperm. MitoSOX Red is a probe developed to quantify selectively cellular and mitochondrial superoxide productions in the mitochondria. MitoSOX Red reagent, oxidized by superoxide, and fluoresce red at 580 nm, can be successfully used in human and bovine sperm).

Sperm chromatin structure reflects the capability of sperm to fertilize the egg and is measurement of the sperm quality. The Sperm Chromatin Structure Assay (SCSA) relies on extend of DNA denaturation which then sperm samples are mixed with an acridine orange (AO), resulting in metachromatic shift from green fluorescence to red fluorescence. In this assay, when AO intercalates with double-stranded DNA (dsDNA) it yields green, but it yields red when it intercalates with single-stranded DNA (ssDNA). Determining the ratio from the mixture of green and red fluorescence, for each spermatozoon, by a 488-nm laser by flow cytometry demonstrates the status of DNA fragmentation (DNA fragmentation index) and the chromatin structure. Also, terminal transferase dUTP nick-end-labeling (TUNEL) can also be employed to evaluate sperm DNA fragmentation by flow cytometry. This assay requires the enzyme, terminal deoxynucleotidyl transferase to catalyze the ration where deoxyuridine triphosphate nucleotides are incorporated into DNA breaks at their 3-hydroxyl ends. TUNEL and SCSA accompanied with flow cytometry have compatibility and produces accurate information related to sperm fragmentation.

Sex sorting is a practical application of flow cytometry which requires applicable protocols and high-speed cytometers. The main principle of this techniques is to determine the DNA content of individual sperms. In this technique, Hoechst 33342 fluorophore is incubated with sperm; it enters the cell and binds to DNA. Because the X-chromosome has a lot more DNA than the Y-chromosome, X- and Y-bearing sperm are separated using flow cytometry. During flow through in the stream, each spermatozoon is enclosed in droplets which are subsequently captured by fluoresce detector. A fluorescence signal from X or Y chromosomes is detected, and positive or negative charge is then assigned to droplets. As they pass through the oppositely charged plate, they are separated into either X or Y tubes consistent with their DNA contents.

There is a need to develop a more comprehensive methodology and novel techniques for assessment of the quality and viability of sperm should be developed or combine new techniques including bioinformatics or mathematical biology with the current techniques to study post-thaw viability. Exploring important aspects of sperm cryobiology, for instance, functional genomics (transcriptomics, proteomics, lipidomics, and metabolomics) and epigenomics (DNA methylation and chromatin dynamics), can have significant positive impact on AI protocols. Novel biomarkers (proteins, small non-coding RNAs such as microRNAs, lipids and small molecules, or epigenomic markers) can be used to better understand spermatogenesis, sperm quality, predict male fertility, and develop better extenders.

10

ARTIFICIAL INSEMINATION IN POULTRY

10.1 INTRODUCTION

Artificial insemination (AI) is the manual transfer of semen into the female's vagina. Basically it is a two step procedure: first, collecting semen from the male; and second, inseminating the semen into the female. In poultry, depending on the objectives and goals of the farm or laboratory, there may be intervening steps such as semen dilution, storage, and evaluation.

Artificial insemination is practiced extensively with commercial turkeys. This is primarily the result of selective breeding for a heavier and broader-breasted commercial turkey and the consequent inability of toms to consistently transfer semen to the hen at copulation. The broiler industry has not adapted AI to the extent of the turkey industry but it is occasionally used in pedigree lines and in regions where labor is relatively cheap.

To grasp the magnitude of AI in the turkey industry compared to that of livestock, a hypothetical flock of 500 breeder hens inseminated with 100 µL of diluted semen (1:1) twice the week before the onset of egg production and once weekly thereafter for the 24 wk of egg production would entail 13,000 inseminations using 650 mL of semen. It should be apparent with these numbers, semen collection and hen inseminations are labor intensive as each male and female must be handled each week.

Looking back over the use of AI in the turkey industry one can safely say that in the 1960s, weekly inseminations were based on semen volume per dose using undiluted semen. In the 1970s and early 1980s, breeder farms began to dilute semen and inseminate a known number of sperm per dose. In the mid-1980s through the 1990s, hens were initially inseminated a week before the onset of lay and inseminations were performed with a known number of 'viable' sperm. Currently, while inseminating before the onset of egg production remains widely practiced, most companies, but not all, have gone back to inseminating a known volume of semen or number of sperm per dose, in the 1970s and 1980s.

10.2. REPRODUCTIVE BIOLOGY OF POULTRY

10.2.1. Overview

The goal of AI is to produce a succession of fertilized eggs between successive inseminations. To accomplish this, weekly inseminations must replenish the sperm population in the uterovaginal junction (UVJ) sperm storage tubules (SSTs). Birds do not have an estrous cycle that synchronizes copulation with ovulation. Alternatively, about 7-10 days before their first ovulation, hens mate, sperm ascend the vagina and then enter the SSTs. At the onset of egg production, individual sperm are slowly released from the SSTs, transported to the anterior end of the oviduct, and interact with the surface of the ovum (see for recent reviews). Whether fertilized or not, over the next 24-26 hr the ovum is transported though the oviduct, accruing the outer perivitelline layer (PL) in the infundibulum, the albumen in the magnum, the shell membrane in the isthmus, and the hard shell in the uterus (also referred to as the shell gland) before oviposition. If fertilized, the blastoderm in the first laid egg consists of 40,000-60,000 cells in the turkey and 80,000-100,000 cells in the chicken.

Ovary: In the hen only the left ovary and oviduct become functional organs. About 2-3 wk before the onset of lay, small (less than 1 mm in diameter) white-yolk follicles begin to accumulate yellow yolk with some being recruited into a hierarchy of maturing yellow-yolk follicles (Figure 1). At the time of ovulation, the largest follicle, designated as F1, is ovulated. About 17 days were necessary for the 1 mm diameter white yolk follicle to mature to a pre-ovulatory 40 mm diameter yellow yolk follicle. After the F1 follicle is ovulated, the next largest follicle, formerly designated F2, becomes the F1 follicle and will ovulate at the beginning of the next daily "ovulatory cycle" in 24-26 hr.

The ovary and oviduct of a turkey hen in egg production occupy much of the abdominal cavity. The ovarian follicular hierarchy consisting of ovarian follicles at various stages of develop (7 maturing follicles visible in this photograph) is observed. The largest follicle, F1 follicle is the next to ovulate. The ovum ovulated about 10 hr earlier has accrued albumen in the magnum (m), a shell membrane in the isthmus, and is observed in the uterus (ut) undergoing shell formation. Its post-ovulatory follicular sheath (POF) appears as an open pocket. The vagina (distal to the uterus and not visible) is embedded in connective tissue and enveloped by the abdominal fat pad.

The follicular sheath surrounding the maturing oocyte consists of histologically distinct concentric layers of cells: the outer serosa (germinal epithelium); the theca externa, which forms the greatest portion of the follicle wall, provides structural support to the follicle and has steriodogenic cells; the theca interna, a highly vascularized layer, which like the theca externa has steroid-producing cells (both thecal layers synthesize androgens and estrogens); and, the granulosa cell layer, enveloping the oocyte, which is responsible for progesterone secretion and the synthesis of the inner PL. The inner PL is homologous to the mammalian zona pellucida and is a fibrous reticulum about 2 μm thick. At ovulation, only the inner PL envelops the ovum. While there is no corpus luteum formation in birds, the thecal layers and the granulosa of the post-ovulatory follicle (POF) produce prostaglandins and progesterone, respectively then regress over the next 72 hr. The POF has a pocket like appearance after ovulation (Figure 1). On the surface of the inner PL overlying the germinal disc (GD), which is a 3.5 mm diameter disc of white yolk containing the haploid pronucleus and associated organelles, are sperm receptors. Sperm bind to the receptors overlying the GD, hydrolyze a path through the inner PL, and are incorporated into the ovum. Polyspermy is normal in birds but only one sperm in apposition to the female pronucleus undergoes nuclear decondensation and initiates syngamy, the reconstitution of the diploid number of chromosomes.

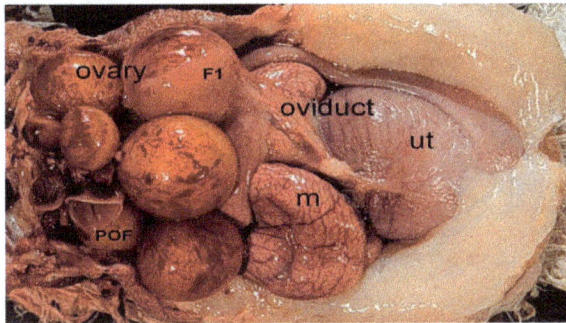

Fig. 1: Ovary

10. 2.2. Oviduct

The mature oviduct consists of five anatomically and functionally distinct segments (Figures 1 and 2): the infundibulum, which secretes an albumen-like product that forms the outer PL and prevents pathological polyspermy; the magnum, responsible for deposition of the albumen proteins; the isthmus, which forms the shell membrane; the uterus (also referred to as the shell gland), a pocket-like structure that elaborates the hard-shell; and, the vagina, which is a conduit between the uterus and cloaca for the egg-mass at oviposition and is responsible for sperm selection and storage following semen transfer. Interestingly, when the vagina and uterus are excised and fixed in toto and the connective tissue surrounding the vagina subsequently removed, the vagina appears as a coiled segment (Figure 3) . This anatomy explains the resistance one feels when performing a vaginal insemination with a straw regardless of the presence or absence of an egg mass in the uterus. If inseminating a hen within 30 min after oviposition, the connective tissue around the vagina and the smooth muscle composing the vaginal wall are flaccid. Venting (exteriorizing the vagina for placement of the inseminating straw) at this time may induce a partial prolapse leading to a deep insemination (closer to the

UVJ) and the forfeiture of sperm selection by the vagina. Such deep inseminations are associated with high embryo mortality, possibly due to pathological polyspermy.

The surface mucosa of each segment of the oviduct is lined with parallel, gently spiraling folds along the longitudinal axis. The surface epithelium lining the luminal mucosa contains varying proportions of secretory and ciliated cells. All segments except the fimbriated region of the infundibulum and the vagina possess sub-epithelial tubular glands that secrete components used in egg formation. However, the anterior 2-3 cm of the vagina, an area referred to as the UVJ (Figure 3), contains the SSTs, the primary sites of sperm storage (Figure 4).

At ovulation, the ovum is grasped by the fimbriated region of the infundibulum and, if sperm are present, the ovum may be fertilized within a 10-15 min interval. Thereafter, infundibular secretions accrue around the ovum, forming the outer PL, which acts as a barrier to further sperm penetration. Birkhead observed that the number of sperm trapped in the outer PL is positively correlated with the size of the ovum and is likewise correlated with the number of sperm that have penetrated the inner PL. Interestingly, the sperm trapped in the outer PL retain an intact acrosome. If fertilized, the first cleavage furrow in the GD appears 7-8 hr post-ovulation, while the egg-mass is in the isthmus.

10. 2.3. Oviductal Sperm Selection, Transport, and Storage

Following deposition in the oviduct, sperm are transported to UVJ by a combination of their intrinsic motility and cilia beat activity. Within the SST lumen, sperm are either widely spaced or oriented parallel with their heads toward the distal end of the SST (Figure 4). Sperm are apposed to, but not directly contacting the apical microvilli of the SST epithelial cells. This spatial relationship may facilitate lipid transfer between the resident sperm and the SST epithelial cells. Interestingly, alkaline phosphatase, known to play a role in lipid transfer, has been histochemically localized in the apical region of the SST epithelium.

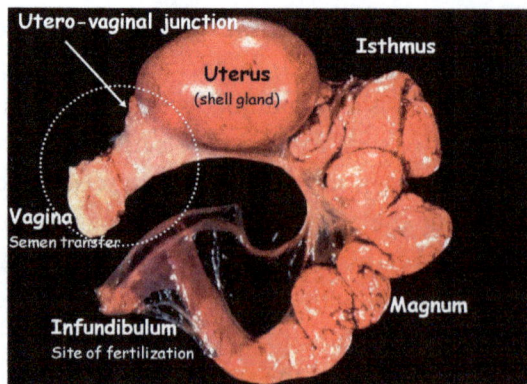

Fig. 2:

The duration of sperm storage in the SSTs is species-dependent. Chickens can store sperm for up to three weeks, whereas turkeys can maintain sperm for 10 weeks in the

SST and still lay a fertilized ovum. This may be related to number of SSTs present in the UVJ; turkeys have been reported to have 20,000-30,000 SSTs, while chickens have been estimated to have only 5,000-13,500. Additionally, after several generations of selection for high fertility, chicken hens possessed increased numbers of SSTs when compared to non-selected control hens, suggesting the number of SSTs may be positively correlated with fertility. In contrast, under commercial conditions, different broiler strains exhibiting different fertility levels revealed similar numbers of SSTs.

The segments of the turkey oviduct with a hard-shelled egg in the uterus are observed. Sperm transferred into the vagina undergo an intense selection process before reaching the sperm storage tubules (SSTs) localized in the utero-vaginal junction. Sperm are slowly released from the SSTs and ascend to the infundibulum, the site of fertilization. In this photograph, the vagina is enveloped by connective tissue.

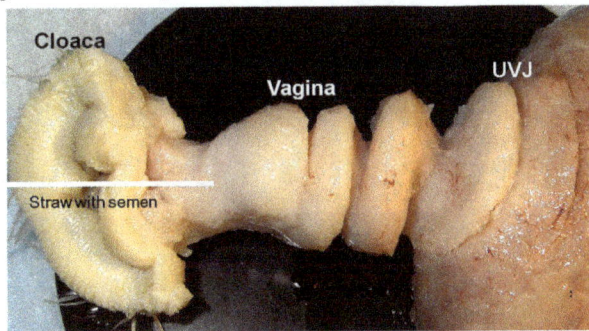

Fig. 3:

Following fixation in neutral-buffered formalin and the removal of the surrounding connective tissue, the coiled morphology of the turkey vagina is revealed. When inseminating a hen, one should insert the straw with the semen until resistance is felt, then release the semen as the straw is withdrawn. As observed here the resistance is due to the coiled vaginal and not an egg mass in the uterus.

Little is known concerning the cellular and molecular mechanisms that sustain sperm within the SST lumen for prolonged periods of storage. These mechanisms likely involve the reversible suppression of sperm motility and metabolism, protection and repair of the sperm plasma membrane, uptake and storage of molecules to sustain sperm metabolism, and maintenance of the SST lumen by removing by-products of sperm metabolism and degraded sperm. It is clear the SSTs generate a discrete environment to maintain sperm viability via the influx and efflux of compounds critical for sperm survival). While ultrastructural analysis has revealed only limited evidence of secretory activity, the identification of membrane-bound vesicles released from the apical tips of the SST epithelial cell microvilli suggests a role in the maintenance of resident sperm through lipid transfer. A large proportion of the sperm plasma membrane is composed of polyunsaturated fatty acids that are highly susceptible to damage induced by lipid peroxidation. The peroxidation of these fatty acids results in increased damage to and permeability of the sperm plasma membrane. A complex system of anti-oxidation enzymes are present in the SST epithelial cells and presumably interact with luminal sperm to minimize damage due to lipid peroxidation and maintain sperm membrane integrity. While many metabolites required by sperm in the SSTs have yet to be identified, increased avidin expression is apparent in SSTs relative to surrounding UVJ epithelial tissue possibly providing a means of sequestering biotin and other vitamins for use by the SSTs or resident sperm. Interestingly, progesterone has been shown to induce expression of avidin in the oviduct, providing a potential link between progesterone fluctuation and sperm storage in and release from the SSTs.

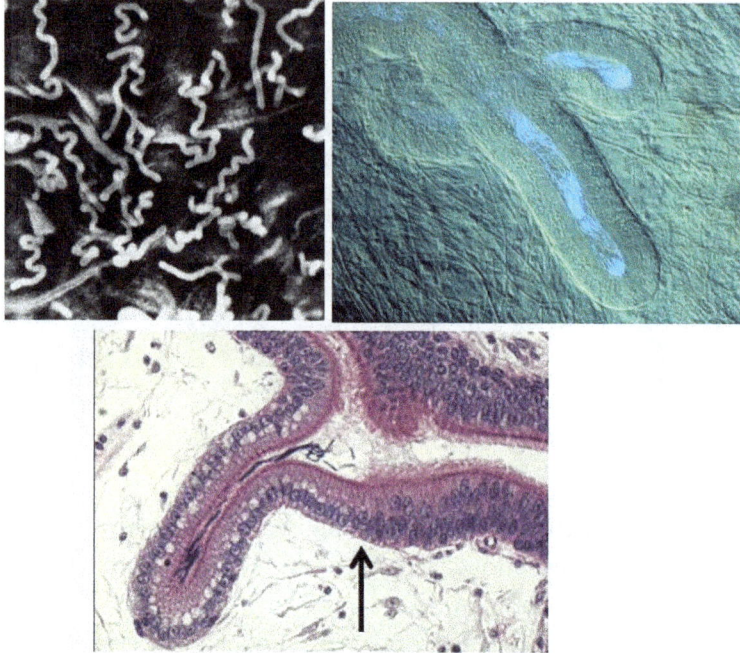

Fig. 4:

Three views of the turkey's sperm-storage tubules (SSTs) are observed. The left panel is a stereoscope image showing the pleomorphic appearance of the SSTs. The length of the SST can be as long as 300µm. In the right panel a hen was inseminated with sperm stained with Hoechst 33342, a nuclear fluorescent dye, the UVJ mucosa containing SSTs was isolated, and an unfixed squash preparation was observed by dual interference contrast and fluorescence microscopy. Sperm with fluorescing nuclei are observed in the two SST lumina. The lower-middle panel shows a histological section of a portion of a SST containing sperm (the dense rod-like structures in the lumen are sperm nuclei. The arrow indicates the transition between the pseudo-stratified columnar ciliated epithelium of the uterovaginal junction and the simple columnar epithelium of the SST that is characterized in histological preparations by the supra-nuclear vacuole.

Sperm exit the SSTs in a slow, continuous stream; however, a stimulus cuing the egress of resident sperm from the SSTs has yet to be identified. The observations that receptors for estrogen and progesterone exist in the SSTs has led to the suggestion that these compounds may trigger release of resident sperm, possibly in response to hormonal cues over the course of the ovulatory cycle. However, an alternate theory suggests the inherent mobility of the sperm plays a larger role than hormonal induction in egress of sperm from SSTs. Resident sperm exhibit a slow, synchronized oscillatory movement in the lumen of SSTs, suggesting the presence of a fluid current through the SST lumen. The identification of water channels, known as aquaporins, in the apical epithelium of SSTs lends credence to a model wherein motile sperm maintain their residence in the SST lumen by swimming against the fluid current generated *via* the aquaporins. In the SST lumen, sperm retain their motility by fatty acid oxidation. It has been suggested the sperm membrane is the source of this fatty acid and that as the quality of the sperm membrane gradually decreases there is a reduction of available ATP and sperm motility decreases. Sperm are then swept out of the SST lumen into the UVJ, where they encounter various stimuli enhancing their motility. These sperm are then transported to the infundibulum, the site of fertilization. Such motility-enhancing factors may include changes in environmental pH and neuroendocrine factors such as serotonin. Further oxidation of sperm fatty acids, possibly sequestered from the surround milieu, generates the energy required for sperm to respond to such motility-enhancing factors and transcend the oviduct.

Once sperm are deposited in the oviduct, several selection barriers must be overcome prior to ascending to the infundibulum and fertilizing an ovum. This selection occurs initially in the vagina: only highly mobile (defined as progressive movement in a viscous medium at 40°C) sperm traverse the vagina. While sperm mobility is a major factor in sperm selection in the vagina, sperm selection is also dependent upon the glycoprotein composition of the sperm plasma membrane. The sperm glycocalyx is highly complex and heavily sialylated and modification of the glycocalyx results in reduced fertility and failure of the sperm to enter the SSTs. Interestingly, removal of membrane-associated carbohydrates did not affect sperm entry into SSTs if sperm were inseminated directly into the UVJ or when co-incubated with UVJ explants, suggesting the glycocalyx plays a central role in sperm transport and selection through the vagina. Further barriers to sperm prior participating in the process of fertilization include sperm release from the SST and subsequent transport to the infundibulum, and their interaction with the ovum.

10.2.4. Sperm: Ovum Interaction And Fertilization

Given the voluminous nature of the hen's ovum and the GD relative to mammalian ova, one must assume that yet-to-be identified factors "attract" sperm to the GD. Examination of the electrophoretic profile of the GD and non-GD regions of the PL revealed no variation in protein composition. Furthermore, the abrogation of the preferential interaction of sperm and the inner PL overlying the GD in vitro suggests the factors underlying the preferential binding of sperm are not necessarily associated with the inner PL. It is clear, however, glycoproteins play a large role in the interaction between the sperm and ova, even if not directly involved in targeting of sperm to the GD in vivo . Pre-treatment of either the PL or sperm with N-glycanases resulted in significantly decreased sperm-ovum interaction in vitro . Conversely, N-linked oligosaccharides released from the inner PL by N-glycosidase treatment could induce the acrosome reaction in sperm in vitro. These findings strongly suggest N-linked glycans, most likely terminal N-acetyl glucosamine residues, have an essential role in the sperm-ovum interaction in avian species, specifically in induction of the acrosome reaction.

Interaction between the sperm and inner PL results in induction of the acrosome reaction. During the acrosome reaction, the inner and outer acrosomal membranes dehisce resulting in the release of acrosin (a trypsin-like enzyme). As the result of the acrosome reaction, sperm hydrolyze a small hole in the inner PL (Figure 5), enabling sperm to reach the microvilli-studded surface of the ovum. The capacity of sperm to hydrolyze and penetrate the inner PL is the biological basis for the sperm penetration assay discussed below and next section.

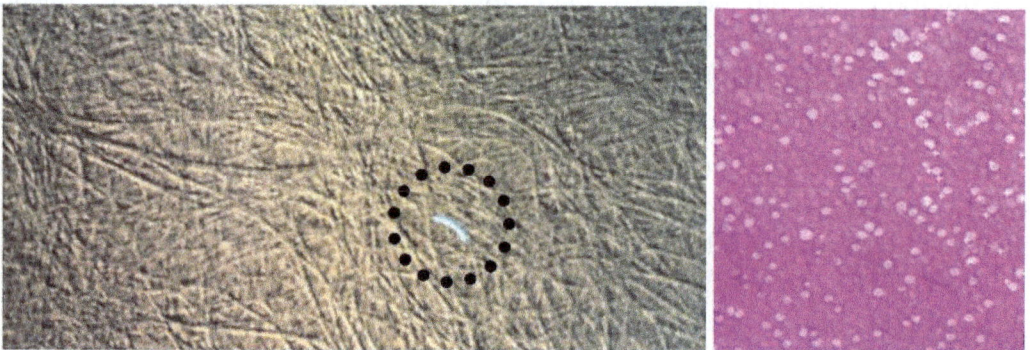

Fig. 5:

In the left panel, a turkey sperm stained with Hoechst 33342 prior to insemination is observed on the surface of the inner perivitelline layer (PL). The sperm's acrosome will release a trypsin like enzyme, acrosin, and digest a hole through the inner PL. The right panel shows multiple sperm holes (white perforations) in the inner PL overlying the germinal disc (GD) of a duck ovum (polyspermy is normal in birds). Sperm hole numbers can be used to assess true fertility and the duration of the fertile period.

Unlike mammals, polyspermy is the norm in avian fertilization. The GD (3.5 mm in diameter) provides a relatively small target for fertilization in the large megalecithal ova (yolk-filled ova) of chickens and turkeys (3.5–4.0 mm in diameter); thus polyspermy may be an evolutionary adaptation to ensure higher rates of fertilization in such species. The inner PL may be penetrated by many sperm, although only one male pronucleus will ultimately fuse (syngamy) with the female pronucleus to form the nascent embryo (reviewed in. A single sperm hole in the inner PL does not ensure fertilization. Although turkeys show a lower number of sperm interacting with ova relative to chickens, the presence of three sperm holes in the inner PL predicts a 50% probability of fertilization, whereas, six sperm holes suggest a probability greater than 95% fertilization. The outer PL is rapidly depositied around the ovum in the posterior infundibulum and proximal magnum and is impenetrable by sperm thus preventing pathological polyspermy.

Given the volume of the GD relative to a single sperm, another possible function of polyspermy may be to activate specific molecular factors in the GD cytoplasm thereby initiating the process of embryogenesis. Yet, polyspermy also results in the presence of multiple male pronuclei in the GD. To cope with this potentially harmful scenario, the mature ovum has been found to have DNase I and II endonuclease activities, both of which will degrade sperm DNA. In contrast, no such DNase activity has been detected in mammalian ova that engage in monospermic fertilization, further suggesting the role of these enzymes in the avian embryo is to protect against detrimental genetic consequences of polyspermy.

The number of holes in the inner PL is highly positively correlated with fertility. Correlations exist between the number of sperm inseminated, the number undergoing the acrosome reaction at the inner PL, and the number of sperm embedded in the outer PL. The number of sperm holes in the inner PL and the number sperm trapped in the outer PL may be used to estimate the duration of fertility ('fertile period') in hens. While the number of sperm penetrating the inner PL shows a decreasing logarithmic relationship over time, a positive correlation between the total number of sperm penetrating the inner PL and the number of sperm stored in the SSTs was observed. Given these observations, it should not be surprising there is also a positive correlation between the number of SSTs containing sperm and the proportion of sperm that have undergone the acrosome reaction at the inner PL.

10.3 TECHNIQUES IN ARTIFICIAL INSEMINATION AND FERTILITY EVALUATION IN POULTRY

For non-domestic birds, chapters in Bakst and Long, Lake and Stewart and Bakst and Wishart provide overviews of semen evaluation and AI techniques. Artificial insemination technology and reproductive biology for ratites were reviewed.

10.3.1. Semen collection

Primarily due to the anatomical variation of the phallic region in different birds, semen collection techniques will vary. In contrast to ratites and water-fowl with an intromittent phallus, Galliformes (chicken, turkey, and quail) do not have an intermittent organ. Their non-intromittent organ consists of folds and bulges that make contact with the female's cloaca at mating. From an anatomical perspective, there are considerable differences between the non-intromittent organs of the chicken and turkey (Figure 6). The rooster has a prominent medial phallic body and relatively small lateral phallic bodies and lymph folds. Conversely, the turkey tom has no medial phallic body but prominent lateral phallic bodies and lymph folds. Sex sorting at hatch by cloacal examination is based on the relative differences in size of these structures between the males and females.

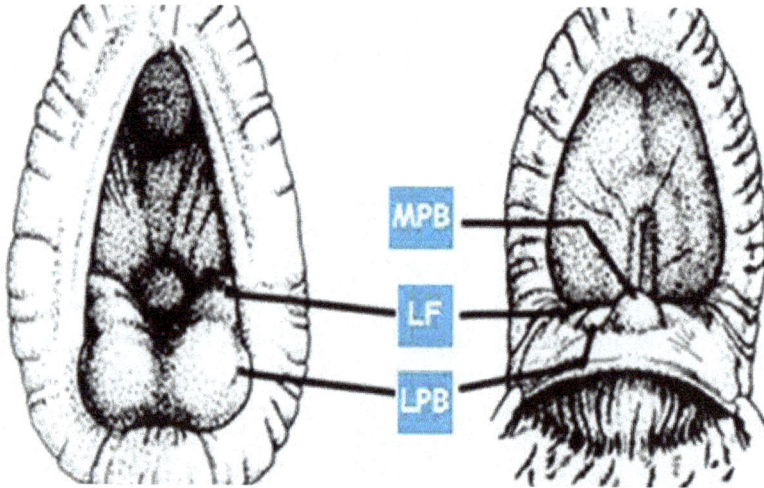

Fig. 6:

The turkey (left) and chicken (right) cloacae are viewed with the dorsal lips of the cloacae pulled back to expose each species phallus non-protrudens. Unlike the turkey, the chicken has a central protuberance, the medial phallic body (MPB) and regressed lateral phallic bodies (LPB) and lymph folds (LF). The turkey phallus non-protrudens is characterized by dominant LPB and LF and the conspicuous absence of the MPB.

The goal of semen collector is to obtain the maximum volume of clean, high quality semen with the minimal amount of handling. In chickens and turkeys, the abdominal massage technique involves massaging the cloacal region to achieve phallic tumescence. This is followed by a 'cloacal stroke', a squeezing of the region surrounding the sides of the cloaca to express the semen. Little additional semen can be expressed after two cloacal strokes; additional cloacal strokes may cause damage to the phallic and cloacal regions and contribute to semen contamination.

Semen should be pearly white, viscous, and clean. With each male collected, the semen collector should perform a visual examination of the semen at the time of ejaculation. This is easier with the turkey because the ejaculate accumulates on the phallus before it is collected by the 'milker' (semen collector). Off-color or watery semen, and semen contaminated with blood or fecal/urates debris should not be used for insemination. Due to the increased volume of transparent fluid in rooster semen, which is a transudate derived from the phallus at the time of ejaculation, chicken semen is less viscous and sperm concentration lower than that of turkey semen.

10. 3.2. Sperm Concentration

If semen is to be diluted, it is best .to have a known volume of semen diluent (a tissue culture-like medium formulated to sustain sperm viability) at ambient temperature in the semen receptacle before collection begins. For routine AI of turkey hens, semen from 10-12 toms are pooled in a single receptacle, mixing the semen gently after each male is collected. Semen volume is determined and if the AI dose is based on numbers of sperm (generally 250-350 million sperm per dose) sperm concentration is determined. The most popular techniques for determining sperm concentration are the packed cell volume (PCV; also referred to as a spermatocrit) and optical density (OD; photometry).

Determining sperm concentration using PCVs is nearly identical to that of determining blood hematocrit values. Semen aspirated into micro-hematocrit tubes are centrifuged in a hematocrit centrifuge until the sperm are tightly packed (10 min); the percentage of packed sperm cells relative to the original semen volume in the micro-tube is determined. Sperm concentration is derived using a conversion factor or standard curve previously derived by comparing and graphically plotting varying ascending sperm concentrations from hemocytometer counts to corresponding spermatocrit readings. (See for detailed protocols to determine sperm concentration and the derivation of standard curves.)

The optical density (OD) is determined using a photometer. The OD of highly diluted semen is directly proportional to the concentration of sperm, thus providing an indirect estimate of the sperm concentration. Like the PCV method, sperm concentration is derived using a conversion factor or previously derived standard curve by comparing and graphically plotting varying sperm concentrations from hemocytometer counts to corresponding OD readings.

The PVC and OD methods are two indirect methods of determining sperm concentration, that is, the final concentration is calculated from a regression equation or standard curve derived, in part, from direct sperm counts with a haemocytometer. Briefly, to derive a regression equation and standard curve, serial dilutions (n=5) covering a wide range of sperm concentrations are prepared and sperm concentrations are determined with a haemocytometer and the instrument or method that requires the standard curve (at least 4 replicates with 4 different semen samples). This is a tedious procedure but if reliable and repeatable sperm numbers are to be inseminated it is best to establish standard curves for each instrument every 12-18 months. The reason for this is that the rotational speed of different centrifuges and the intensity of a photometer's light source may differ as a result of manufacturer's variation, age of the instrument, and/or repeated use of the instrument, thereby producing variations in the respective final readings and subsequent calculations of sperm concentrations.

Another concern when using any semen evaluation method is variation in the operator's techniques. Consistency is the key to repeatable data. The technical staff all must follow the same standard operating procedures (SOPs). For example, when counting sperm with a hemocytometer, all individuals in a lab should following the same SOP for how long the sperm are permitted to settle on the grid and which sperm to count or omit from the count. Also, is the photometer zeroed with the same buffer? If a procedure calls for an incubation period, such as in a live-dead stain, are the samples being incubated for the same duration each time using the same stain concentrations? A lack of consistency in following the SOPs within a laboratory will lead to unwarranted variation and non-reproducible and inaccurate data.

10.3.3. Sperm Viability

In the context of semen evaluation, reference to 'viable' sperm simply implies that such sperm possess an intact plasma lemma and are assumed to be functional. Plasma lemma integrity is frequently determined using either a dead-cell or a live-cell stain alone or simultaneously. The dead-cell stains are excluded by sperm with an intact plasma lemma but stain dead sperm possessing a permeable plasmalemma. Live-cell stains permeate the intact sperm plasmalemma and become visible only after reacting with cytosolic enzymes or interacting with sperm nuclear proteins. Both eosin and propidium iodide are popular dead-cell stains while calcein AM and SYBR-14 are frequently used live-cell stains (see for extended discussion and availability for the live-cell probes). On a commercial breeder farm, the nigrosin/eosin (N/E) technique is most likely the procedure to be used to determine sperm viability. Briefly, sperm are stained with N/E and a smear of the stained sperm is made on a slide (Figure 7). Under a bright field microscope the viable sperm remain pearly white, while eosin will stain non-viable sperm a pink to magenta color. The nigrosin serves as a background to enhance differentiation between the non-viable and viable sperm. In contrast to the N/E technique, a more sophisticated laboratory may use flow cytometry that sorts viable from non-viable sperm after staining with calcein AM or SYBR-14 and propidium iodide.

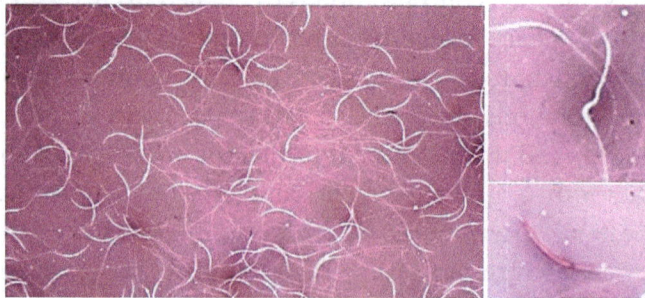

Fig. 7:

The left panel shows a nigrosin eosin preparation of turkey sperm with nearly 100% viable sperm (unstained) white nuclei and midpieces. The sperm head is clearly visible as the white arcing segment; the acrosome and midpiece are difficult to differentiate from the nucleus. The upper right panel reveals a normal sperm and a second sperm with an abnormally curved and swollen midpiece. Observed in the lower right panel is a nonviable sperm stained with eosin throughout the nucleus and midpiece. Barely visible at the anterior end of the nucleus is the unstained, conical shaped acrosome.

10.3.4. Sperm Motility and Mobility

Sperm motility can be progressive (forward direction) or non-progressive (random movement or oscillations) movement. Generally, progressive motility is determined subjectively at ambient temperature using a microscope at low magnification (hanging-drop technique) or objectively using a computer-assisted semen analysis system. These techniques are reviewed by Bakst and Long. Motility evaluated by microscopy has been shown to have little correlation with fertility and simply reveals that the sperm are motile. First described by Froman and McLean and further elaborated for commercial use by Froman, the sperm mobility assay has gained popularity as a measure of an individual male's ability to produce highly mobile sperm [mobility defines the ability of sperm to move progressively against a viscous medium that are more likely to fertilize an ovum than males producing less mobile sperm. While the sperm mobility assay is a powerful tool for the selection of the most fecund males to be used in AI, it necessitates attention to details and accurate and consistent preparation of the reagents.

10.3.5. Evaluation of Fertility

The measure of a successful AI program is sustained hen fertility. While candling-fertility is useful, there is an eight or more day lag between the last AI and candling-fertility determination, which overlaps with the next insemination (hen insemination is generally at 7-day intervals). With AI programs, it is often desirable to determine the fertility status of a flock before the next weekly insemination. There are several options available: breaking-out fresh eggs and examining the GD to differentiate a fertilized from an unfertilized or early dead embryo; setting normal but culled eggs (checked, hairline cracked, or dirty eggs) in a spare incubator for 24-36 hr before breaking-out; counting sperm in the outer PL; and counting sperm holes in the inner PL. The above procedures are reviewed in Bakst and Long.

As noted previously, the sperm penetration assay is not only used to determine true fertility, but also to estimate the number of sperm residing in the use SSTs at the time of ovulation. The isolation of the inner PL and staining procedure, initially developed for chicken eggs, was quickly adapted to turkey eggs. The major drawback to the sperm penetration assay as originally described is that it is time consuming, particularly with respect to isolating, washing, and positioning the PL wrinkle-free on the slide. Spasojevic and colleagues at Willmar Poultry Company (Willmar, MN) significantly increased the efficiency of preparing the PL slides from turkey eggs in the following manner: the albumen is removed from the ovum as in the original procedure; a square is outlined on a slide using super glue; the slide is placed firmly on the ovum's surface with the GD centered in the square; after the glue is set, the PL is cut and washed to remove adhering yolk. The advantages here are speed and the PL remains wrinkle free.

A different modification of the sperm penetration assay was suggested by I.A. Malecki (personal communication) and entails placing a filter ring over the GD (inside diameter slightly larger than the GD), cutting around the outside diameter of the filter ring (about 2 mm between the inside and outside perimeter of the ring), and lifting the filter ring off the ovum. The filter ring with the adhering PL is washed gently with saline to remove the yolk and GD material until transparent, placed on a slide, and then fixed and stained with saline washes after each step. Our laboratory has used the filter ring technique with eggs from broilers, turkeys, ducks, and quail and it is now our preferred method for the performing the sperm penetration assay.

10.4 ARTIFICIAL INSEMINATION IN POULTRY: AT A GLANCE

Artificial insemination is a common practice in the poultry industry with the turkey industry in North America and Europe using it almost exclusively for the production of hatching eggs. The broiler industry has not adapted AI for several reasons: because of sheer numbers of broiler breeders that need to be inseminated weekly, the labor cost would be very significantly; the initial investment in special housing for the males; an efficient, cost effective means of actually performing the inseminations (housing and catching the hens) would need to be developed; and finally, the concern that after a few generations of breeding broilers by AI, the behaviors associated with natural mating may be less dominant. Notwithstanding these concerns, the benefits of AI for broilers would include the following: the male:female ratio would be increase from 1:10 for natural mating to 1:25 with AI; with fewer males needed, there would be greater selection pressure on the male traits of economic importance and subsequently greater genetic advancement per generation; biosecurity concerns associated with "spiking" aging hen flocks with new and/or younger males to augment mating frequency and fertility would be eliminated; and, differences in body conformation between males and females that impact semen transfer at mating would no longer be a consideration.

In 1995, Sir Peter Lake wrote an excellent review of the history of AI, its impact on the poultry industry, and what is needed to advance the practice of AI with poultry. Unfortunately, AI technology has not advanced significant since this review article. More than 15 years later, the only significant advance is in the evaluation of sperm mobility and the impact that males producing highly mobile sperm have on paternity. Notwithstanding, it is foreseeable that sometime in the future, research addressing poultry sperm biology and the cellular and molecular basis of oviductal sperm transport, selection, and storage will lead to the following innovations in AI technology: insemination intervals increased to 10-14 days (versus 7-day) with fewer sperm per insemination; *in vitro* sperm storage for 24-36 hr at ambient temperature with minimal loss of sperm viability; and, the possibility of transgenic progeny following the insemination of sperm carrying transgenes.

11

LAPAROSCOPIC ARTIFICIAL INSEMINATION TECHNIQUE IN SMALL RUMINANTS

11.1 INTRODUCTION

Assisted reproductive technologies (ART) are utilized in animal reproduction to promote efficient use of germplasm for improvement of genetic value of companion and production animals. Artificial insemination (AI) is one such ART that has revolutionized the cattle breeding industry within the past few decades. With development of more efficient methods of semen cryopreservation and estrus synchronization, it is now possible to obtain higher pregnancy rates even with poor quality frozen semen via artificial insemination. Unlike cattle though, the small ruminant semen industry in the US is unorganized and semen testing and cryopreservation parameters are not rigorously implemented. There is a growing demand for use

Laparoscopic artificial insemination (LAI) is an intrauterine method of insemination, especially utilized in the small ruminant species to bypass their unique anatomically tortuous cervix. There are several advantages of LAI that include efficient use of processed semen leading to higher pregnancy rates. Success of LAI programs depends on proper implementation of estrus synchronization programs, patient selection and thorough knowledge of the reproductive physiology.

of frozen and processed semen especially in the show lamb industry, where owners are willing to pay a premium to introduce newer genetics in their flocks. However, ewes/does bred with frozen or processed semen typically have a lower pregnancy rate when bred via conventional methods such as vaginal (VAI) and trans-cervical artificial insemination (TCAI) techniques. This is due to the long and tortuous nature of the cervix in small ruminants and the presence of 4–7 cervical rings. These cervical rings point caudally into the lumen thus providing a physical barrier to attempts at passing an insemination pipette during TCAI. There is ample evidence that pregnancy and lambing rates improve as the depth of semen deposition in the cervix increases. The degree of penetration of the insemination pipette through the cervix depends on the breed, age and stage of the estrous cycle especially in ewes. Deeper semen deposition results in greater numbers of motile spermatozoa available for fertilization thus leading to higher pregnancy rates.

Laparoscopic artificial insemination is an advanced assisted reproductive technique that enables such deep intrauterine deposition of semen and helps bypass the physical barriers of the caudal reproductive tract in small ruminants. Pregnancy rates using frozen semen deposited intra-uterine via laparoscopy have yielded higher pregnancy rates (60–80%) consistently when compared to vaginal and TCAI methods. In addition to higher pregnancy rates, it is possible to use lower concentrations of spermatozoa per breeding thus leading to more number of animals bred per ejaculate. The average dose required for breeding a ewe using frozen semen can be as less as 20–25 million live spermatozoa, when compared to higher doses required via the vaginal (400 million live spermatozoa) and trans-cervical route (100–200 million live spermatozoa). Thus, a single entire frozen ejaculate can be used to inseminate as many as 50 to 100 ewes, thus leading to a more efficient use of semen. The main disadvantage of providing LAI service to producers has been the high equipment cost and the relatively steep curve of surgical expertise required to perform to perform the procedure safely. However, with the availability of newer and more portable laparoscopy equipment, it is now possible to offer these services cost-effectively at a hospital and field setting.

11.2 MATERIALS REQUIRED

Most equipment and associated costs quoted here are from the manufacturer Karl Storz®, Germany, though there are other manufacturers available in the market as well.

    a. Trocars and Cannulas—There are two common sizes available that suit the purpose (i) 10 mm and (ii) 5 mm. Estimated cost $500.

    b. It is preferable to use the smaller size as there are several advantages: (i) Enables creating smaller incisions and ports, (ii) Lesser chances of abdominal perforation due to lesser effort required during insertion (iii) Lesser wear and tear of instruments, (iv) No need for trocar adaptors for AI guns (v) Enables use of smaller rigid 5 mm telescopes (laparoscopes).

    c. Telescope/Laparoscope (available options are 0 and 30°): We prefer using a 0°scope, but a 30° oblique telescope can also be used effectively. Estimated cost $7,000 (new)—$3,500 (refurbished).

    d. Light Source with halogen/xenon bulbs and cables: Approximate cost around $7,000.

There are handheld portable endoscope light sources available now which are better suited for field work and just as effective costing around $500.

    a. Video camera and screen (optional, since many practitioners in a field setting prefer looking through the lens of the laparoscope instead of using a camera and screen). Approximate cost $3,500–4,000.

b.   A new mobile video-endoscopy unit available from Karl Storz® known as the Tele Pack Vet X Led® is multifunctional and contains a camera, light source; air insufflation unit and image capture capabilities. This unit is light, portable and can be carried out to the field in a carry case (provided). It can also be adapted for concurrent use in small animal and equine clinical practice. Approximate cost $25,000.

c.   Air insufflation unit—A medical grade air insufflation unit with carbon dioxide tank can be used to ensure an ideal abdominal pressure. However, the equipment is expensive and cumbersome to move around especially when performing this procedure at a field level. Also, the rate of insufflation is relatively slower leading to increased surgical time and increased duration of the patient in a Trendelenburg position. Instead of a traditional air insufflation unit, a regulator can be attached directly to the CO_2 tank which enables faster insufflation. The disadvantage is that the degree of insufflation is subjective and based on abdominal percussion and degree of distention. Yet another alternative is to use a commercial vacuum pump system (e.g., GAST® vacuum pump) with an attached inline filter. The advantage of using such filter systems is that besides CO_2, other alternative gases such as medical grade air or room air can also be used for insufflation. Disadvantages of using room air are that it is risky to use in a dusty environment due to the danger of causing peritonitis. A recent research study has shown that there is no danger of hypoxia or infections in using medical grade air vs. CO_2 Nor were there any differences in pregnancy rates observed between the two groups. In a hospital setting we prefer to use the vacuum pump and insufflate with room air. We have performed more than 400 surgical procedures using room air, without any reports of complications such as peritonitis or septicemia. There were no differences found in pregnancies rates with use of room/medical air as compared to CO_2.

d.   Medical grade air insufflation unit: $8,000, C_2 tank with regulator: $250, Commercial vacuum pump (e.g., GAST® Mfg.): $500.

e.   Laparotomy surgical pack: We recommend having ready access to a laparotomy surgical pack, for the purpose of isolating and suturing any subcutaneous bleeding vessels after the LAI procedure or for performing an emergency laparotomy in case of an abdominal organ perforation.

f.   Laparoscopy AI cradle: These are specialized cradles that can be tilted almost up to 90° to position animals in a Trendelenburg position. We recommend buying cradles with aluminum frames as they are sturdy yet light to transport in case of field work (Sydell® Iowa, Minitube® USA etc.). Approximate cost: $1,500.

Semen Processing:

⊙   AI guns and sheaths: Transcap with guide (IMV®, France): $550; Aspics for semen straws: $70/25 pcs; Robertson's AI gun with sheaths (Minitube® USA): $500.

◉ Semen processing equipment: Semen tube holders, semen straw thawing equipment, slide warmer, portable microscope, 0.25 cc straws, straw cutters etc. (Total cost around $3,000 including the microscope).

11.3 LAPAROSCOPIC AI PROCEDURE

11.3.1 Selection of Patients

LAI though minimally invasive is still a surgical procedure nonetheless and hence young, healthy ewes/does in appropriate body condition scores (BCS's) are ideal candidates for the surgery. It has been shown that an optimum BCS results in higher ovulation as well as pregnancy rates. Fat/obese animals not only prove to be a surgical risk, but also may not respond appropriately to synchronization protocols (AI or Embryo transfer), thus increasing the net surgical procedure time. A decrease in embryonic viability and subsequently lower pregnancy rates have been observed in animals maintained on a body score of below 2 and above 4. The proposed mechanism behind pathogenesis in overly conditioned animals has been attributed to lower progesterone levels possibly because of increased liver blood flow, leading to increased clearance of the hormone from circulation. The preparation of animals for estrus synchronization and LAI begins several weeks prior to actual date of the procedure. This involves vaccinations, deworming and increasing the plane of nutrition (flushing) to achieve an ideal BCS. However, in a recent report the pregnancy rates declined in ewes handled 4–6 weeks prior to LAI for various managemental procedures such as deworming, vaccinations and feet trimming. A possible explanation to this decreased pregnancy rate was attributed to the stress experienced during such procedures. Hence, special care in terms of minimizing stress should be undertaken when handling animals for routine preventive managemental procedures. In addition, attention should be paid to detect the presence of systemic diseases in the flock such as infections of the respiratory system which increases surgical risk to the affected animal. The estrus synchronization protocols are sent out several weeks prior to the day of the procedure. A thorough knowledge of reproductive physiology, seasonal and breed variations, appropriate duration of protocols and drug dosages are essential for adequate response from patients. Shorter protocols can be designed for animals that are cycling and during breeding season, whereas out of season protocols tend to be longer in order to prime the inactive reproductive tract for estrus. Older animals that have undergone surgical embryo transfers or multiple LAI procedures in the past can have

Proper equipment and surgical expertise help in reducing patient morbidity and mortality rates. LAI can be associated with several complications as a result of inadequate patient preparation, poor technique or equipment failure. Hence, a thorough planning is essential to carry out the procedure safely and with consistent success rates. Addition of LAI to a small ruminant/food animal practice can be quite profitable and professionally fulfilling, as long as an appropriate investment in equipment and adequate training of veterinarians and technical staff is implemented.

extensive adhesions of the omentum to the parietal peritoneum thus forming a curtain/ barrier or, in some cases adhesions to the reproductive tract. This can lead to difficulties in visualization of the reproductive tract and increases the duration of surgery or the need to abandon the procedure halfway. Based on the reproductive history, animals suspected of being pregnant should be checked via trans-abdominal ultrasound examination before initiating the synchronization protocols. Since the LAI procedure involves restraining animals in a Trendelenburg position, it is recommended to keep the animals off-feed for at least 16–20 h and off-water for at least 12 h to prevent abdominal fill and minimize chances of regurgitation and aspiration.

11.3.2 Sedation and Premedication

Light sedation is usually recommended since the total duration of the procedure (preparation and surgery) takes roughly about 10–15 min only. The goal is to have the patient stand up on their feet after they are loaded off the cradle and start searching for food.

Two classes of drugs that we recommend for sedation are alpha-2-agonists (Inj. Xylazine@ 0.05–0.1 mg/kg of the 20 mg/ml large animal formulation I.V. or I.M.) and tranquilizers (Acepromazine@ 0.05–0.1 mg/kg I.V. or I.M.). Opioids such as Butorphanol (0.05–0.2 mg/kg IV, IM, SQ) may also be used 5 to 10 min before handling animals for restraint. The advantage is that they afford some degree of analgesia, but personal experience has shown that it also leads to lesser degree of sedation than alpha-2-agonists, causing more struggling among patients when they are restrained in a Trendelenburg position. Other medication such as anti-inflammatories and in some cases long acting antibiotics (Ceftiofur crystalline free acid or Long acting Oxytetracycline- extra label usage) can also be administered during restraint and surgical preparation. Local analgesia in form of Lidocaine hydrochloride is administered at each proposed incision site (2 ml of 2% Lidocaine hydrochloride subcutaneously) and each site is scored with a hypodermic needle to mark the area for future reference. An appropriate withdrawal time for meat and milk should be relayed to the producer when using any of the above drugs.

11.3.3 Pre-Surgical Preparation

The patient (ewe/doe) is restrained and sedated with the appropriate sedative agent and observed for clinical effects. Once adequate sedation is confirmed, the animal is then lifted and restrained on a special, custom made laparoscopic AI cradle. The fore- and hind-feet (at level of hocks) are restrained securely, a face mask or a towel is used to cover the eyes and the animal moved to the surgical-prep station. The wool on the ventral abdomen is clipped from the level of the mammary glands and extending cranially up to the umbilicus. The area is surgically scrubbed with 2% Chlorhexidine scrub alternating with 70% isopropyl alcohol. Special attention is to be paid to the inguinal gutters as they accumulate loose dirt, dried feces, natural sebaceous secretion, and which tend to contaminate the surgical site when the animal is suspended in a Trendelenburg position. Two sites about a hands width cranial to mammary glands and adjacent to the left and right mammary/superficial epigastric veins are identified. The site can be medial or lateral to the veins and the choice is dependent on the preference of the surgeon and size of the patient. For larger patients (>120 lbs.), we recommend a more medial approach since the abdomen is wide and tends to get wider when insufflated with CO_2/air. This prevents the laparoscopic instruments from reaching the reproductive tract or aligning with each other during the insemination process. On smaller patients (< 120 lbs.), a more lateral approach is recommended to afford adequate insufflation and avoid more medially placed abdominal organs. The surgical sites thus selected are superficially scored with a 20 G-1-inch needle, and 2 ml. of 2% Lidocaine hydrochloride infiltrated in the subcutaneous tissues and musculature (Figure 1). The skin scoring is performed to identify the surgical sites during surgical procedure, since the local anesthetic tends to dissipate quickly. A final surgical scrub is performed before wheeling the patient to the surgical station.

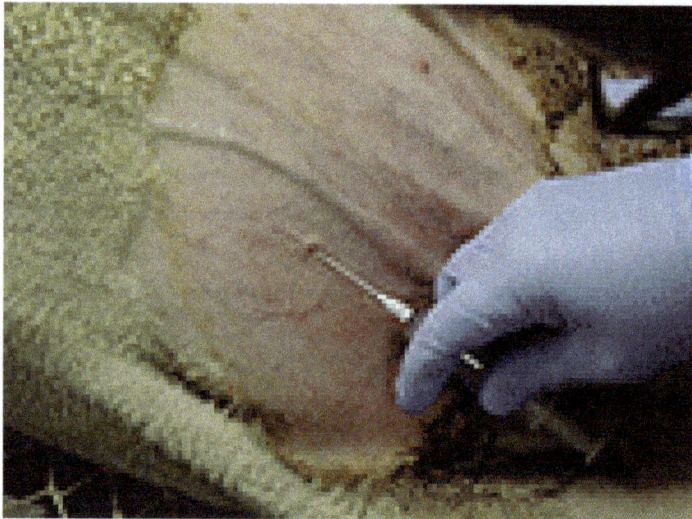

Fig. 1: Surgical sites are located cranial to the udder and medial or lateral to the mammary/superficial epigastric veins. Local anesthetic is infiltrated, and the sites are scored to identify them prior to the surgical procedure. Left of the image is cranial.

11.3.4 Surgical Procedure

The LAI cradle is elevated up to 45°, to position the ewe in a Trendelenburg position. A no. 11 scalpel blade is used to create 0.5 inch incisions through the skin and fascia up to the level of muscle over the proposed pre-scored incision sites. A 1.5-inch blunt teat cannula attached to a sterile flexible insufflation hose is inserted pointing laterally through the muscle layers and intra-abdominally via the incision farther from the surgeon with a firm, calculated push. Air insufflation is carried out till the ventral abdomen feels adequately tense. With practice it is possible to carry out LAI with lesser amounts of air safely. The advantage of insufflating lesser amount of air is to reduce the degree of hypoxia to the patient while in Trendelenburg position. A 5 mm trocar and cannula are inserted in the abdomen through the near incision with calculated pressure (Figure 2), the trocar withdrawn, and a 5 mm Telescope/Laparoscope inserted via the cannula to visualize the interior of the caudal abdomen. The reproductive tract (uterine body and horns) are usually located ventral (from a surgeons' point of view) to the urinary bladder. In animals that have responded adequately to estrus synchronization protocols, a distinct tone and hyperemia can be identified affecting the reproductive tract. The tract appears pale to dark pink and responds by curling when it is touched by the laparoscopic instruments (Figure 3). The location of the tract and its relation to surrounding structures is noted to ascertain the ease with which an intra-uterine injection can be performed safely. On some occasions, a distended bladder can hide the reproductive tract partially or completely. Decompression of the bladder during premedication and surgical preparation is strongly recommended to prevent this from happening. The caudal sac of the rumen, distended cecum or loops of small intestine can sometimes prevent visualization of the reproductive tract. This can be minimized by keeping the patient off feed and water as recommended. Once the reproductive tract is visualized, another similar sized trocar and cannula is inserted adjacent to the teat cannula. A loaded laparoscopic AI gun carrying a 0.25 cc semen straw with an external sheath (IMV®, France) is then inserted through this port and aligned opposite the greater curvature of uterine horns under laparoscopic guidance. The external sleeve/guide can be used to manipulate the uterine horns from underneath overlying structures such as the bladder or omentum to the desired angle. The Aspic and needle apparatus is then exposed keeping them as close to the uterine horns as possible and with a quick jab the needle is seated at the level of the mid-horn. Semen can be injected either in one or both uterine horn as per the operator's preference (Figure 4). Where a single 0.25 cc straw is to be utilized per breeding we prefer injecting both horns with half the straw of semen. However, when a 0.5 cc straw (divided in two aspic guns) is available for use per insemination, an entire gun can be injected per horn. Care is to be taken to ensure proper depth of the needle placement while inseminating to prevent semen leaking in the abdomen. There are no reported advantages of injecting both horns, and the entire dose can be deposited in one horn only, resulting in similar pregnancy rates. However, when performing LAI procedures in animals superovulated for embryo recovery, it might be beneficial to inject both horns so that adequate numbers of spermatozoa are available on both sides for migration and fertilization in presence of increased intrauterine mucus due to higher circulating estrogen levels. In addition, injecting both horns also serves as insurance if there is leakage of semen from or incomplete insertion of the lumen at one injection site.

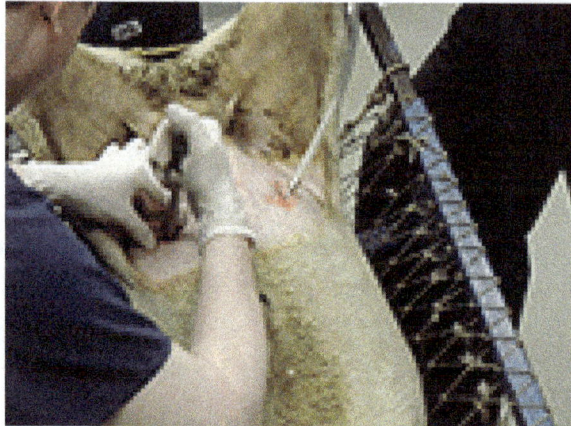

Fig. 2: A 5 or 10 mm trocar and cannula pointing laterally, are inserted through the near incision into the abdominal cavity with a firm pressure and the trocar withdrawn to be replaced with a laparoscope.

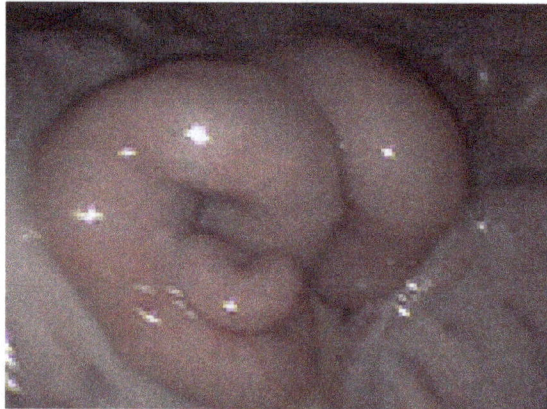

Fig. 3: Intra-abdominal view of the reproductive tract. The uterine horns have a distinct tone and color under the influence of estrogen. This type of appearance is classified as Grade 2.

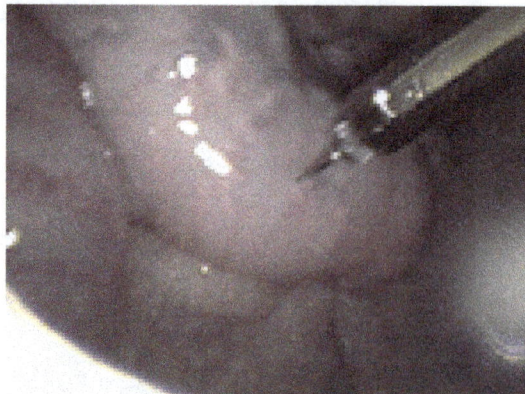

Fig. 4: A laparoscopic AI gun and needle apparatus are used to inject semen intra-uterine at the level of the mid-horn along the greater curvature.

Once the uterine horns are injected, a quick assessment is made to ascertain that there is no excessive bleeding or uterine horn lacerations. The laparoscope and the AI gun are withdrawn from the cannulas. The spring loaded or side valves are decompressed to deflate the abdomen and the animal is lowered to a horizontal plane after removal of all instruments from the abdominal ports.

The skin incisions are closed with the help of non-absorbable suture material (Prolene® 2-0, Ethicon®, USA) in a cruciate suture pattern after ensuring that there is no excessive bleeding. On occasion, subcutaneous branches of the mammary/ superficial epigastric veins may bleed excessively. The bleeding vessels are clamped and ligated individually and then the skin incisions closed in an interrupted suture pattern. Skin staplers can also be used and are faster to apply but can be costlier than suture material. We prefer to cover the abdominal incisions with a water resistant antibiotic free aluminum based wound spray (Aluspray®, Neogen® Animal Safety, USA). We also prefer administering a reversal agent in case alpha-2-agonists were used for sedation (e.g., Tolazoline, Yohimbine) as soon as the animal returns to a horizontal plane. Most animals stand up immediately or at least assume a sternal recumbency after being placed on the ground. In cases of prolonged lateral recumbency it is advised to monitor the animal's vital signs closely and prop the animal in a sternal position to avoid aspiration pneumonia.

11.4 COMPLICATIONS ARISING DURING LAPAROSCOPIC AI PROCEDURE

As with any surgery, there are numerous complications that can arise during the LAI procedure.

11.4.1 Complication Arising During Insemination of Systemically Unhealthy Animals

One of the major concerns when carrying out LAI is patient mortality due to underlying systemic disease conditions such as respiratory tract infections. A thorough history and physical examination of preferably each animal (when dealing with small groups) is crucial in order to avoid identifying these unhealthy patients. Each animal should be thoroughly observed and checked for signs of coughing and wheezing, especially evident when handling or segregating animals in different groups or during premedication. Despite taking due care, there may be animals that are missed, raising the percent morbidity and mortality rates. Minimizing the surgical procedure time greatly helps in reducing chances of such complications, and is largely dependent on surgical speed and efficient teamwork which is gained through practice. Judging the tone and color of the reproductive tract greatly helps in assessing whether the patients have responded adequately to estrus synchronization protocols. For patients that have poorly responded or not responded at all (flaccid, pale tract) to the hormonal protocols, a decision can thus be reached quickly to abandon the insemination process early enough during surgery. It is always important to constantly monitor vital parameters and signs for regurgitation from the nose/mouth to prevent aspiration pneumonia. Flow-by oxygen via face mask can also help in lessening the degree of hypoxia experienced during the procedure. In animals that are obese or metabolically compensated, we advise the owner against performing the procedure, or decreasing angle of elevation from 45 to 30° after insufflating the abdomen. This reduces pressure on the diaphragm and lessens the degree of hypoxia experienced during the surgical procedure.

11.4.2 Rupture/Puncture of Abdominal Viscera

The abdominal organs in danger of being punctured are the urinary bladder in the caudal abdomen, small intestinal loops and cecum in the mid-abdomen and caudal sac of the rumen in the cranial abdomen (Figure 5). To minimize the risk of perforation there are a few things to be kept in mind before and during the surgical procedure:

- Ensure that the animals are adequately fasted and kept off-water.
- Ensure that the urinary bladder is emptied/decompressed to minimize chances of perforation
- Proper and adequate insufflation of the abdominal cavity.
- Proper placement of the trocars: The surgical sites for trocar placement (as described before) should be meticulously selected. Too cranial a site can result in perforation of the caudal sac of the rumen. Too median a placement can result in mammary vein punctures, urinary bladder ruptures, cecal, and small bowel perforations. While placing the trocars through the proposed surgical sites it is also important to angle them laterally. Using smaller trocars (5 mm) also enables for easier insertions through the body wall. The larger 10 mm trocars can create a considerable drag leading to greater force required for insertion and subsequently greater risk of perforation of abdominal organs.

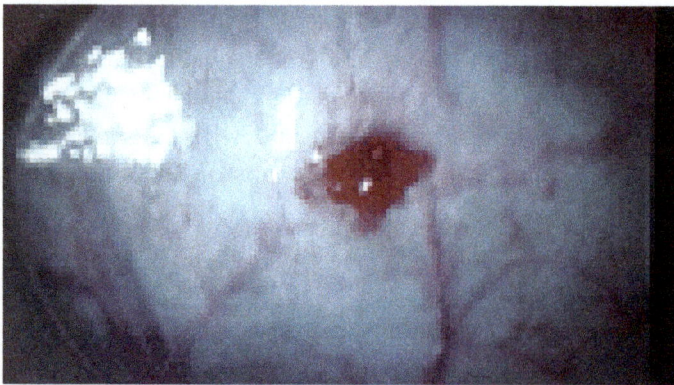

Fig. 5: Abdominal organs such as the rumen and the cecum are frequently in danger of rupture during trocar placement especially if the animals are inadequately fasted. The following figure shows a cecal rupture due to insufficient duration of feed and water withholding.

One of the early signs of a possible gastrointestinal tract perforation is methane like odor evident from the cannula immediately after removal of the trocar. The trocar may have greenish-yellow fecal contents stuck on its end and along the shaft. Bladder ruptures should be suspected with presence of a sudden increase in blood tinged fluid evident in the abdominal cavity (Figures 6, 7). Most ruptures can be confirmed on direct visualization of the organ. However, on some occasions the sudden deflation of a distended viscus can change shape and orientation of the affected organ thus preventing confirmation by direct visualization. On rare occasions, rupture of a major blood vessel such as the aorta or its branches can lead to excessive bleeding and sudden death.

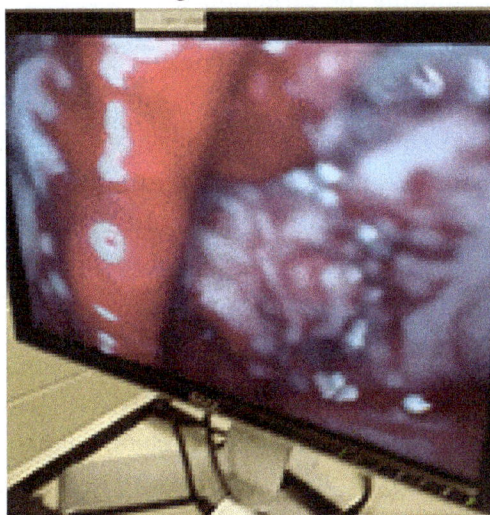

Fig. 6: Iatrogenic bladder rupture during trocar insertion due to inadequate decompression prior to surgery.

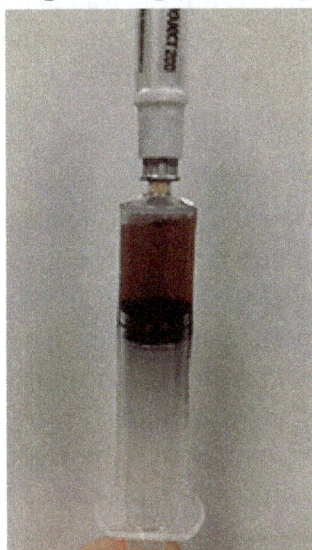

Fig. 7: An abdominocentesis post-iatrogenic bladder rupture revealing tan colored fluid consistent with urine.

11.4.3 Subcutaneous Emphysema

In larger animals having a broad abdominal girth there is risk of subcutaneous emphysema developing if the trocars are placed too laterally. This disrupts the normal tissue planes and increases risk of the trocar getting caught between different layers of the abdominal wall, making it difficult to enter the abdominal cavity. In cases of subcutaneous emphysema, the air insufflation needs to be stopped immediately and the leaked air gently massaged out of the incision site. If addressed early, the same site can be utilized for trocar placement. But if a significant amount of subcutaneous air is present, it is best to select another surgical site after suturing the earlier port.

11.4.4 Abscess Formation/Peritonitis/Sepsis

A small percentage of animals in the flock may develop peritonitis, external or internal abscesses, sepsis and death. This usually happens when contaminated instruments are used without cleaning them between animals. We recommend dipping and thoroughly wiping off the instruments using 70% alcohol or dilute 2% Chlorhexidine solution, after each surgery and before they can be used for another animal.

11.4.5 Hematoma/Subcutaneous Bleeding

Due to the proximity of surgical site to branches of the mammary/superficial epigastric veins, it is possible to accidently incise a collateral branch leading to excessive subcutaneous bleeding. The blood can leak into abdominal cavity coating laparoscopic instruments and blurring the visual field. Presence of blood can also lead to formation of intra-abdominal adhesions in future. Post-surgery, these vessels can continue bleeding in the subcutaneous tissue leading to formation of a localized hematoma. Since the clotted blood and fibrin are a good media for bacteria to thrive, this can lead to formation of an abscess. After the abdomen is deflated and laparoscopic instruments withdrawn, the surgical sites should be meticulously checked for presence of small bleeding vessels. These should be ligated before suturing/stapling the incision sites.

11.4.6 Intra-Abdominal Adhesions

In animals having undergone LAI procedures or surgical embryo flushes in the past, intra-abdominal adhesions of the omentum to the body wall can form. These result in a partial or complete division of the abdominal cavity thus making it difficult to align laparoscopy instruments through the two opposite ports. Efforts to maneuver the instruments around the adhesions or sometimes injecting through the omental barrier are the only options available. On occasions creating three abdominal ports or creating ports on the same side of the body can help circumvent around these adhesions. Sometimes incomplete insufflation can lead to the omentum getting caught on end of the laparoscopic instruments (Figure 8). Adequate insufflation of the abdominal cavity usually results in the omentum falling off instruments affording a clear view of the abdomen.

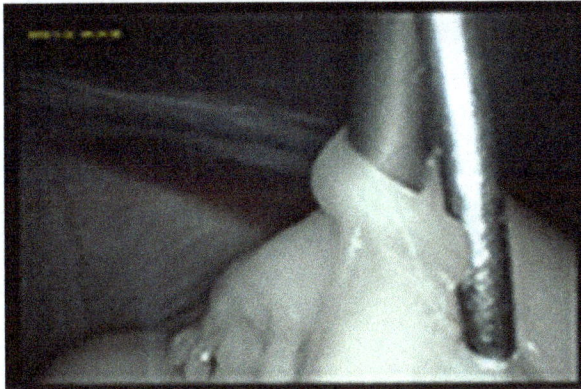

Fig. 8: The omentum and omental fat can sometimes get entangled with the laparoscopic instruments due to insufficient insufflations. This can prevent visualization of the reproductive tract and other abdominal contents.

11.4.7 AI Gun Failure

Sometimes the AI guns may get stuck due to faulty "O" rings or due to faulty batch of semen straws. On occasion, because of "O" ring failure, the injecting straw can disengage and fall in to abdomen (in case of Aspic straws, IMV®) increasing the risk of abdominal organ perforation due to the exposed injection needle. Hence, a laparoscopic grasping forceps should be included in the LAI surgery pack to address such complications. It is always a good idea to load an AI gun with a mock straw filled with saline before start of the procedure to ensure that all parts of the instrument are working well.

11.4.8 Inability to Seat the Injection Needle in the Uterine Lumen

In cases where the animals fail to respond adequately to synchronization protocols, the AI gun needle may slip out of the uterine musculature because of the lack of uterine tone. Owners should be informed about such lack of response, the AI process stopped and the animal resynchronized. We document the color and tone observed for each animal during the surgical process. This provides us and the owner a valuable feedback when observing for pregnancy rates and infertility problems in the flock. The uterine tone is graded as: Grade 0—No response; Grade 1- medium degree of response (Figure 9); Grade 2—adequate/good response (Figure 3). The color can vary from pale to different shades of pink depending on stage of estrus. There has been no difference observed in pregnancy rates between Grade 1 and Grade 2 uterine tone and color based on a recent retrospective study conducted by the author and colleagues (unpublished data). The uterine horn increases in thickness during superovulation protocols as compared to conventional AI protocols, and hence a marginally longer aspic injection needle should be used to ensure the proper intraluminal deposition of semen.

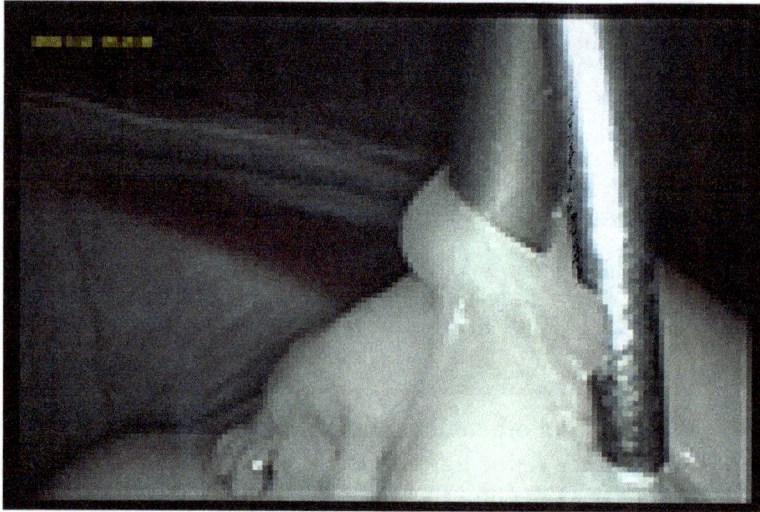

Fig. 9: Grade 1 uterine tone and color showing a relatively pale uterus with minimal tone.

11.4.9 Uterine Bleeding

The uterine tract in estrus has increased blood supply; hence a little oozing from the injection sites is expected. To minimize extensive bleeding or prevent uterine vessel lacerations, it is advisable to inject along the greater curvature of the uterine horns. The lesser curvature which is close to the broad ligament has a rich vasculature and is prone to bleed extensively if injected (Figure 10).

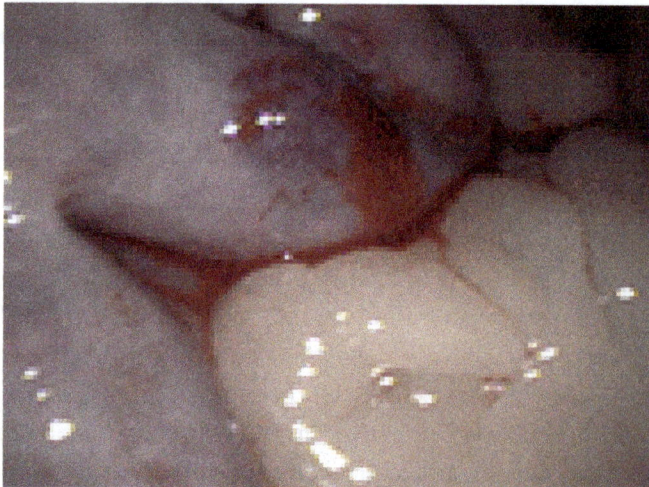

Fig. 10: Accidental injection of semen along the medial or lesser uterine curvature can cause bleeding and hematoma formation due to the extensive vasculature in the broad ligament.

The most common complications observed are hypoxia in over conditioned animals, subcutaneous bleeding, omental adhesions from prior surgeries and localized hematomas.

On rare occasions, we have observed perforations of the gastrointestinal organs (in unfasted animals) and the urinary bladder. These usually occur during trocar placements, thus highlighting the importance of feed/water withdrawal and bladder decompression prior to conducting the procedure.

11.5 LAPAROSCOPIC ARTIFICIAL INSEMINATION: AT A GLANCE

LAI involves a substantial investment in form of buying equipment and training for the procedure. The success of LAI program requires a good team work and coordination. A trained veterinarian performs the LAI, a trained technician/assistant handles semen processing and other personnel take part in handling, sedating and prepping animals for surgery. On occasion, producers and owners can be trained adequately to prepare animals for the surgery. It takes a few attempts for the team to get used to the flow of the procedure. However, once the operator and the team become proficient with the process, it is possible to inseminate as many as 100–200 animals per day. Addition of LAI to your small ruminant private practice can thus be an economically feasible option that can turn profitable quickly, once producers see an increased pregnancy rate even with use of processed semen.

12

PROBLEMS OF ARTIFICIAL INSEMINATION IN DROMEDARIUS CAMEL-FAILURE OF OVULATION

12.1 INTRODUCTION: AN OVERVIEW

Artificial insemination (AI) is a well accepted method used to achieve faster genetic improvement in livestock species. This has been developed to its optimum extent in cattle and buffalo, while in some other domesticated species of livestock, including the camel, it is yet to be developed. AI is claimed to have been highly successful in Bactrian camels (ARTHUR, 1992), but in dromedary camels results have been less encouraging. Workers at the Camel Reproduction Centre, Dubai have claimed pregnancy rates of 50-60% with fresh diluted semen used within 30 minutes of collection, but conception rate decreased dramatically to 25-30% if semen was not used for 24 hours. All the pregnancies were established with a particular extender and no pregnancy could be established with frozen thawed semen). Likewise, pregnancy results from almost nil with diluted-chilled/frozen-thawed semen to 40% with whole semen have been reported in India (DEEN et al., 2003). The reasons for poor success have not been determined but a major difficulty with AI in camel is to ensure ovulation in inseminated animals. It also observed that the incidence of ovulation and pregnancy is significantly lower in female camels inseminated either with fresh undiluted or diluted semen alone than those obtained with AI following mating with vasectomised teaser. MUSA et al. (1992) opined that deposition of 1 ml of fresh semen, or else exogenous administration of hCG, is essential to ensure ovulation. Entrapment of spermatozoa in thick viscid camel semen (BROWN, 2000) and its speculated role as a sperm reservoir in the female genital tract also need to be considered. *In vitro* extension of semen and its storage could hinder the protective role of this natural reservoir to the spermatozoa in female genital tract.

Camel is an induced ovulator and it has a short luteal phase in non-pregnant female camels (AGARWAL et al., 1991). ARTHUR (1992) reported that unmated and anovulatory camels have basal progesterone levels, those which ovulate but do not conceive show a peak value of 6-10 days after mating, which declines to baseline by day 12. A high progesterone concentration beyond day 12 after mating is a very strong indication of pregnancy. Thus, peripheral progesterone profiles of individual female camels after AI may enable the detection of ovulation, fertilization and pregnancy, which in turn may provide an insight into the possible causes of low success of AI in this species and pave the way for further courses of research to strengthen this technique. With this objective in mind progesterone profiles of inseminated female camels were monitored to assess status of ovulation, fertilization and embryo survival in these females.

An artificial insemination study was conducted on 17 female camels which were administered human Chorionic Gonadotrophin (hCG) to induce ovulation after confirming a follicle in the ovaries using sonography. The animals were inseminated with either diluted-cooled or fresh undiluted semen. No female camel could be impregnated with diluted and cooled semen, while pregnancy rate was low with neat undiluted semen. To ascertain possible causes of low conception rate, plasma progesterone (P4) profiles were monitored. Criteria adopted for interpretation of these profiles were as follows: P4 levels below 1 ng/ml on days 5-8 was considered to indicate failure to ovulate; a single peak of 1ng/ml on days 5-8 followed by a decline on day 12 was considered to indicate ovulation. However, failure of fertilization and P4 levels of more than 1 ng/ml on days 5-8 and day 12 followed by a decline was considered to indicate successful ovulation and fertilization, but failure of embryo survival. Consistently higher levels of P4 were considered to be indicative of pregnancy. Using these criteria, 5 of 33 inseminations were diagnosed as pregnant, while profiles of 17 of 33, 8 of 33 and 3 of 33 were indicative of failure of ovulation, failure of fertilization and failure of embryo survival, respectively. A high incidence of failure of ovulation may be due to oversized follicles or follicles in which degenerative processes might have been initiated prior to administration of hCG. High failure of fertilization may be due to a viscous form of camel semen, which may play a role as a sperm reservoir and protect the viability of spermatozoa in the female genital tract by entrapping sperm. Insemination with diluted and cooled semen may disturb the protection, resulting in failure of conception. It is concluded that the high incidence of ovulation failure and failure to deposit sperm in its natural entrapped viscous form are the major problems for development of AI in the camel. Further improvement may be expected, if we are able to standardize the appropriate insemination time around peri ovulatory time, and appropriate follicular size, which responds to hCG.

12.2 METHODS USED

Thirty-three female camels proposed for experimental artificial insemination were subjected to routine screening for ovarian follicles using pie scanner-200 ultrasound machine and trans-vaginal transducer of 5 MHZ capacity (Pie Medical equipment B.V. Philipsweg, The Netherlands) The camels were sedated with 100 mg of xylazine (Iziner, Intaas Pharmaceuticals, India) administered intravenously while restrained in a sitting posture. Those females which exhibited mature ovarian follicle of 15-20 mm or greater in diameter were injected intramuscularly with 5000 IU of hCG (Profassir, Serono, Italy). The animals were inseminated 24-48 hrs after injection either with cooled semen, frozen thawed semen or with whole semen. Tris egg yolk (FOOTE, 1970) glycerol was used to extend the semen. Semen was extended initially at a rate of 1:1 with unglycerolated diluent and then a final dilution to 1:3 with glycerolated dilutor within 30 min of collections. The semen samples were packaged after extension into labelled plastic cryovials of 2 ml capacity, which were placed in a glass beaker containing water (25 °C) for cooling in a refrigerated unit to 4 °C within 2 hrs. They were then further maintained at this temperature for another 3 hrs.

Freezing of semen was carried out in an automated liquid nitrogen based programmable freezer KRYO 10-1.3 (Planer Products Limited, U. K.) using the protocol of ALMQUIST (1969) developed for dairy cattle, which is as follows:

- Start temperature   4 °C
- Cooling Rates
- From 4 °C to -15 °C   -1 °C per min
- From -15 °C to -60 °C   -4 °C per min
- From -60 °C to -100 °C   -20 °C per min

Finally, the cryovials were plunged and stored in liquid nitrogen until required. Thawing was accomplished by immersing the vial containing frozen semen in a water bath at 40 °C for 2 minutes. Post-thaw motility examinations were accomplished using thermostatic stage inverted phase contrast microscope (Nikon).

Artificial insemination. The female camels were restrained in a sitting position and sedated with xylazine 100 mg i v (Izine·, Intaas Pharmaceuticals, India). For inseminations using diluted semen, a hard plastic catheter was passed per vagina to the cervix and then manipulated by recto-genital palpation into the uterus. Six ml of semen (1:3 extension) was inserted through the pipette into the uterus with a syringe. For whole semen (3-5 ml) deposition, a 20 ml syringe was used. Blood samples were collected by jugular venepuncture in heparinized vials on days 0, 3, 7, 10, 14, 17, 21, 24, 28 and plasma was separated in a refrigerated centrifuge (C- 24, Remi, India) at 2500 rpm. Plasma samples were preserved at -20 °C until used for P_4 analysis. Progesterone analysis of plasma samples was conducted with Coat- A- Count RIA kits (PITK PG-1, 2002-12-11) of Diagnostic Products Corporation, Los Angeles, CA 90045-5597. Inter- and intra-assay coefficients of variations were 5 and 7.5%, respectively, and minimum detection limit was 0.1 ng/ml.

Ovulation, fertilization and pregnancy were determined through progesterone profiles using the following criteria: anovulatory camels had basal progesterone levels (less than 1 ng/ml), while those that ovulate, but do not conceive, exhibit peak values (more than 1 ng/ml) at 6 to 10 days after mating, which then declines to baseline by day 12. Those camels which ovulate and conceive show P_4 values >1 ng/ml on both days 6-10 and day 12. Early embryo loss was suspected when progesterone profiles declined to basal levels after day 12, while pregnant camels show elevated progesterone concentrations throughout gestation and were also confirmed to be pregnant by rectal palpation. Mean ± SE on progesterone profiles on different days were calculated for each group, and chi-square test was applied. 12.3

12.3 EXPERIMENTAL RESULTS

Results are presented in Table 1 and Fig. 1 in the form of a line diagram. Fig.1 shows mean progesterone profiles of all 4 groups of female camels. Series 1 comprised mean progesterone values indicative of luteal phase. All these animals were confirmed clinically pregnant, completed their gestation and delivered healthy calves. Series 2 comprised a mean progesterone profile of 17 female camels, which exhibited levels below 1 ng/ml, indicating failure of ovulation. Series 3 comprised progesterone profiles of 8 female camels, which showed only two points above 1 ng/ml. These levels indicated ovulation but failure of fertilization. Series 4 comprised mean progesterone profiles of 3 female camels, which showed higher profiles at more than 2 points, followed by a decline. These levels indicated successful ovulation and fertilization, but failure of embryo survival. Based on these results, the low conception rate in AI in camel can be categorized and rated as follows:

Failure of ovulation 17/33 (51.51%)

Failure of fertilization 8/33 (24.24%) and

Early embryonic death 3/8.

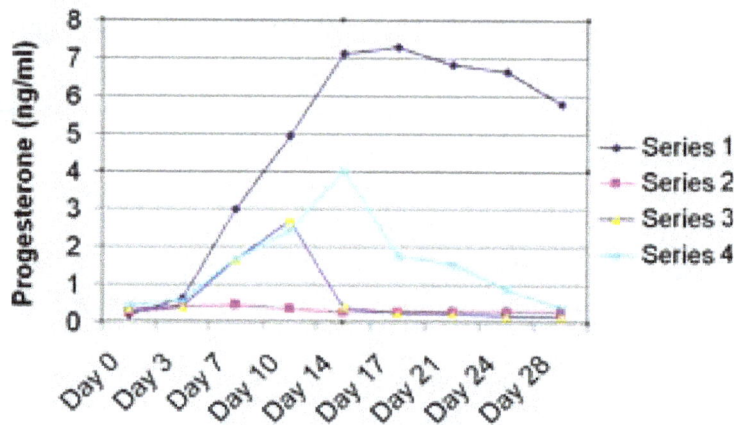

Fig.1: Progesterone profiles of artificially inseminated female camels

Table 1. Mean ± SE of progesterone profiles of artificially inseminated female camels grouped as pregnant, failure to ovulate, failure to fertilize, and early embryonic deaths

Group	Days, progesterone (ng/ml)								
	0	3	7	10	14	17	21	24	28
Chi-square value significance	-	-	ns	s	s	s	s	s	s
Pregnant	0.19 ± 0.06	0.63 ± 0.18	2.99 ± 0.78	4.94 ± 0.57	7.12 ± 1.48	7.28 ± 1.25	6.83 ± 1.72	6.64 ± 1.32	5.80 ± 1.21

Failure to ovulate	0.25 ± 0.04	0.4 ± 0.06	0.46 ± 0.06	0.35 ± 0.05	0.28 ± 0.03	0.27 ± 0.03	0.29 ± 0.04	0.29 ± 0.05	0.29 ± 0.03
Failure to fertilize	0.32 ± 0.12	0.42 ± 0.07	1.66 ± 0.52	2.70 ± 0.75	0.39 ± 0.08	0.26 ± 0.05	0.23 ± 0.04	0.19 ± 0.05	0.17 ± 0.05
Early embryonic death	0.44 ± 0.19	0.58 ± 0.13	1.69 ± 0.72	2.45 ± 0.64	4.01 ± 1.51	1.78 ± 1.36	1.57 ± 1.44	0.89 ± 0.54	0.39 ± 0.10

ns - nonsignificant, s - significant

Chi-square test on mean values of peripheral plasma progesterone profiles indicated significant differences in four groups of camels, viz. pregnant, failure to ovulate, failure to fertilize and early embryonic deaths.

12.4 AT A GLANCE

Since the female camel is an induced ovulator and ovulates only after mating with a male camel, it becomes essential to induce ovulation in AI program by exogenous administration of hormones (MUSA et al., 1992) or by mating with vasectomised teaser[F. Mating with a teaser is considered not to be practical due to the potential spread of venereal diseases. Exogenous administration of hCG or GnRH is preferred to induce ovulation. However, despite exogenous administration of hCG, success rates are

It is concluded that failure of ovulation has been the major factor responsible for low conception rates in artificial insemination in the present study. Size of follicle needs to be monitored prior to administration of hCG. Those greater than 18-20 mm must be avoided in order to improve ovulation rate. Another important factor, which must be considered, is the viscosity and gel form of semen, which seems to serve as a sperm reservoir in the female genital tract and has some protective action on the viability of spermatozoa. These problems need to be resolved if AI has to be developed in this species.

not high, as observed in the present study, where 51.51 % female camels did not ovulate. Similar problems of ovulation in inseminated female camels were reported by ANOUASSI et al. (1992), who observed ovulation in only 33 and 20% of female camels, which were inseminated with raw or diluted semen, respectively, as compared to 60% in those mated with a vasectomised teaser. This problem of anovulation needs to be resolved if AI is to be developed in this species. The size of the follicle at the time of administration of hCG and AI is reported to play an important role. In general, 83-85% of the females were reported to ovulate after breeding if the diameter of the existing follicle was between 13 and 16 mm. Ovulatory response to treatment with hCG, GnRH or mating was reported to be highest when the size of the dominant follicle was between 10 and 22 mm, while follicles that were larger than 22 mm might have already begun a degeneration and may not respond to treatment . Also reported as many as 35-45% to 50% anovulatory follicles. It is possible that poor ovulation response in the present study could have been due to oversized follicles which might have begun degenerative changes prior to treatment. Thus, improvement in efficiency can be possible by selecting appropriately sized follicles prior to treatment. Additionally, exact mechanism of ovulation in this species also needs further investigation. Chinese workers in particular held the view that a GnRH-like hormonal factor is present in seminal plasma and initiates ovulation, while, others could find no such evidence of injection of whole semen, seminal plasma, water or prostaglandin in the release of sufficient LH from the pituitary gland to cause ovulation. Mechanical stimulation of the cervix has also been found not to hasten ovulation in the camel. As such, the ovulatory response in the camel could be the result of a combination of stimuli, including a chemical factor in the seminal plasma, neuro humoral response to the mechanical stimulation of the coitus, and the male effect. Ovulation and pregnancy rates were significantly higher in inseminated camels which had been mated by a vasectomised male. Further investigations on the role of the male in inducing ovulation, particularly poll gland secretion, may be helpful in devising appropriate measures to improve ovulation efficiency.

In the present study, the pregnancy rate with refrigerated diluted semen was nil. Successful impregnation of female camels could be possible with deposition of whole semen only. Successful pregnancy with frozen thawed semen was reported only in Bactrian camel by Chinese workers. In fact, they reported pregnancy rates of 87-91%, which is much higher than would be expected, even from natural mating. Moreover, no repetition of such successful application in other parts of the world has been reported. For example, no pregnancies have been reported to date after inseminating the dromedary camel with frozen semen; pregnancy rates of 50-60% have been reported in camels inseminated with fresh diluted semen within 30 minutes of collection. Conception rate decreased to 25-30% in camels inseminated with semen cooled and stored for 24 hr. Moreover, all the pregnancies were achieved with cooled semen diluted in Green buffer (IMV) + 20% egg yolk only. Also observed very poor pregnancy rates in small camelids, which could be improved using whole undiluted semen. Successful impregnations of female camels with undiluted semen, and no success with diluted chilled semen, indicate some important seminal factor. Camel semen was formerly used in gel form, and spermatozoa are entrapped in gel. Entrapment seems to play a vital role similar to that of a sperm reservoir in other species. Dilution of semen with extenders and in vitro storage might disturb the reservoir form of function and protective action of semen gel on sperm viability, which may be responsible for failure of impregnation with frozen thawed and cooled- stored semen.

13

CRYOPROTECTANTS & CRYOPRESERVATION OF EQUINE SEMEN

13.1 INTRODUCTION

No one can argue that artificial insemination (AI) has not changed the practice of animal reproduction. Artificial insemination has provided the means of:

⊙ Taking a single male ejaculate and breeding numerous females,

⊙ Transporting genetics without the necessity of the movement of animals,

⊙ Limited the risk of injury during mating and

⊙ Limited the transmission of disease.

Equine semen is a one of the most difficult in the industry to cryopreserve efficiently without causing damage to the membrane or apoptosis. This review consists of an in depth analysis of current cryoprotectant classes, membrane damage issues, reactive oxygen species generation, and apoptosis- all of which are exacerbated by cryopreservation.

However, early efforts to incorporate AI into production schemes were limited by the functional lifespan of ejaculated spermatozoa. Therefore, widespread the use of AI Cryopreservation (CP) is the ability to store cells and maintain their integrity and viability at a sub-zero temperature until needed. Like some of the greatest discoveries, CP of semen was the result of a fortunate lab error. In 1949, Ernest John Christopher Polge and his colleagues were focused on trying to use sugars as cryoprotectants (CPO) using what they thought was a stock fructose solution. Polge's research was the beginning of a formidable industry, and decades later we are still striving to make improvements.

13.2 OVERVIEW

The year 1957 was monumental for CP of equine semen, as Canadians, Barker & Gandier reported the first foaling using frozen epididymal spermatozoa,[2] demonstrating use of the technique was possible in the horse. However, this early success has not led to widespread use of the technique as it has in other industries, due to the unique nature of equine semen. Ultimately, not only will the specificity of the species play a large role, but each individual's own body chemical composition may impact the process as well. Cryopreserved equine semen faces differences in at least two areas: the physiological and biochemical components of the spermatozoa themselves, and variations in the anatomy and physiology of sperm transport in the female reproductive tracts. Currently, stallions generally do not fit the protocols of freezing programs due to the unsatisfactory post-thaw sperm quality and fertility rates.4 The quantitative differences seen in the required number of spermatozoa necessary for insemination between species is a largely important element when looking at the potential fertility of cryopreserved semen, and if there are a larger number spermatozoa required for insemination this means there can be less tolerance of poor freezers and poor survival rates. In the horse, the accepted number of viable spermatozoa for insemination is more individual dependent than in other species. Studies have consistently shown CP sperm lack in motility, viability and intact membranes when compared to that of fresh semen. Hence, in the horse, the development of successful freezing procedures will involve more than the identification or application of novel CPO's and additives.

Motility remains a major criterion used to determine the success or failure of a new freezing procedure, but this is contradictory since motility does not positively correlate with the sample's future fertility. On the contrary, the classical definition of a "successfully preserved sperm cell" requires they have the ability to fertilize an oocyte, and to produce a viable embryo via AI. Using this definition, frozen/thawed sperm cells must be able to undergo capacitation, activation of the enzymes within the acrosomal cap (while in the female tract), which allows the sperm cell to penetrate through the zona pellucida and fertilize the oocyte.

Cryopreserved stallion sperm exhibits a high degree of male-to-male variability with respect to cell viability after thawing. In order to adequately classify the quality of frozen semen there must be an understanding of the relative classification of a "good" or "poor" freezer. These concepts are based on post-thaw motility characteristics, including percentages of progressively motile sperm and velocity rate. Tischner proved that only about 20% of the stallions exhibit "good" semen freezability with parameters being more than 40% progressively motile sperm post-thaw. "Fair" freezing stallions post-thaw with 60% motility, and progressive motility range of 20-40%. "Poor" quality semen has a <20% survival whereby with a post-thaw progressive motility rate of less than 20%.

It is generally accepted that even under the best of conditions that 40-50% of the sperm cell population will not survive CP even with optimized protocols.[7] In some species (including the horse) and specific individuals' survival rates can be much lower, making them self-impeding to use of the CP process. Given the known limitations, Vidament accepted stallions showing a post-thaw motility greater than 35% and sperm exhibiting 'rapid velocity', while Loomis & Graham accepted stallions with a post-thaw progressive motility greater than 30%. Ultimately, these collaborative efforts have led to the commercially acceptable semen quality post-thaw of 30% progressively motile sperm, however even then there are many stallions that do not meet this standard. Previous studies have evaluated membrane structure characteristics, and suggested, in some cases, there may be genetic detriments, predisposing the cell to certain survival issues under CP stress; supporting the concept of individuals being classified as "good or "bad" freezers. By developing an understanding the classes of "good" and "bad" freezing semen, patterns can be established allowing the modification of the components of CPA that permit the further improvement of this area of ART by suggesting which medias are more beneficial for each class and will produce optimal results.

13.3 CRYOPROTECTANTS

Semen is highly individualistic, as no two stallions have the same chemical composition, and therefore each will freeze differently. Some individuals have been known to be hypersensitive to glycerol, whereas others may be able to tolerate it well. Following industry demands, a wide variety of CPO's as well as many different commercially available CPA's, have been developed. The current consensus is that CPO's work by minimizing exposure to osmotic stress, stabilizing biomolecule and structure, and limit the effects of reactive oxidative species (ROS). The ideal CPA would not osmotically dehydrate the cell or induce cryoinjury and it would be non-toxic. The goal of a CPO should be to minimize intracellular freezing, minimize cell damage due to the freezing environment and promote cell survival upon thawing. Larger amounts of CPA concentrations, have be shown to lead to more cellular damage; since cells exposed to those penetrating solutes undergo intense initial dehydration, then rehydration, resulting in a chance of gross cellular swelling to occur when the CPO is removed. Ultimately these radical changes in volume and size can lead to damage and death of the sperm.

13.4 CPO CLASSES

There are two classes of CPOs: penetrating and non-penetrating which when used together, increase the cells' chance at survival while reducing the cellular water content to help prevent intracellular freezing.[7] Penetrating agents are micromolecules, which permeate through the plasma membrane of the sperm cell. Acting intracellularly, penetrating agents replace cellular water, as it pushed to the extracellular region, ultimately preventing internal ice crystal formation that could potentially rupture the membrane. Examples of penetrating agents would include DMSO, glycerol, methylformamide (MF) and dimethylformamide (DMF). Non-penetrating agents or macromolecules, capitalize on their increased concentrations within the extracellular regions during the first phase of freezing, generally -10 to -20°C, where they osmotically extract water from the cells.[7] Some non-penetrating agents worth noting include: egg yolk, sugars, liposomes, milk proteins and polymers that can form extensive hydrogen bonds with water. CPO is generally a combination of penetrating and non-penetrating agents each of which has a specific role in aiding the survival of the sperm cells during the freeze/thaw process.

13.5 GLYCEROL

The used of glycerol as a CPO for stallion semen was first described in 1950, by Smith & Polge. This formulation, remaining virtually unchanged, has be the mainstay of the freezing industry ever since.[14] It has been noted as the most effective CPA for lowering intracellular water freezing15 while providing osmolality adjustments to the CPO via invasive thermal protection.[16] Research to understand the mechanisms of CPA led to the discovery of glycerol's' effectiveness in its ability to prevent various phase transitions while freezing via increased water permeability and fluidity of the sperm membranes. However, while glycerol has allowed the CP of numerous species, it may not be ideal CPA. Results in cattle have shown a loss of fertility with aged sperm. Further, while glycerol serves as the leading CPO for many species that was not the case for the equine species. While glycerol provides satisfactory protection for the roughly 20% of animals classified as "good freezers," it has proven detrimental to remaining 80% due to its heavy viscosity and molecular weight. Additionally, glycerol has been shown to be toxic to non-frozen sperm and have contraceptive effects on mares.

Initial studies linked glycerol with the stabilization of semen membranes, by its ability to cause a fluid to gel transition, however this finding led to the expectation of higher CP survival rates. However, recent research has demonstrated glycerol induces cellular damage during the freezing process and, in addition to cryoinjury, could be a largely contributing factor to poor post that motility and fertility rates. While the nature of semen glycerol toxicity is not fully known, some data suggests its use may lead to protein denaturation, directly altering the plasma membrane and the disrupting actin interactions. Further, even though glycerol is a penetrating agent, it is extremely slow in permeating the plasma membrane, which induces osmotic stress which may be the ultimately cause of its toxicity. A number of studies have demonstrated that the addition and removal of glycerol is an important factor responsible for the reduction on post-thaw motility and viability of horse sperm. Equine spermatozoa have been shown to have a limited osmotic tolerance. Glycerol has been shown to induce more distinct osmotic stress with more severe alterations on motion variables, cell viability and acrosomal integrity.

The issues with glycerol toxicity have led to the research and testing of countless other penetrating CPA's, with the idea of finding one that will be less toxic, while yielding comparable or better quality results. This new era of CPO bases include combinations of penetrating CPA, for example glycerol and dimethylformamide. Early results suggest these combinations have lower molecular weights, increased water solubility and minimal toxicity, all of which have proven to advantageous to the preservation of the delicate chemical composition and plasma membrane structure of stallion semen.

13.6 DIMETHYLSULFOXIDE

DMSO is a sulfur containing, organic molecule, which easily crosses cellular membranes. The fast penetrating capacity of DMSO helps to decrease the amount of time necessary to displace water from the intracellular fluid to the extracellular environment. Given the variability seen in stallion sperm, a small amount of this strong compound is often used in conjunction with glycerol or another CPA as an added speed component, and to help stabilize the cell prior to freezing. However with some species DMSO is favored, and used in much larger proportions than necessary for livestock. Species, whose semen specifically perform better following freezing with DSMO may do so because glycerol acts as a contraceptive for them. A few species that have benefited from DMSO as a primary CPA include: mice, rabbits and a variety of fish-including: zebra fish, carp broodstock, seven-band grouper[24] and mutton snapper. Rabbit sperm appear to do best with a substantial proportion of DSMO in relationship to glycerol for CP. Some research suggests this could be do the lack of water channel protein Aquaporin 7 (AQP7), which coincidentally serves as a glycerol transporter.21 DMSO has also been used for semen CP in some members of non-human primate family. Two species, both part of the macaque family: Cynomolgus monkey (Macaca fascicularis) and Rhesus Monkey (Macaca mulatta), have shown mixed results. The Cynomolgus semen was successfully frozen when DMSO was in an equal concentration to glycerol, whereas the Rhesus was unsuccessful after using a stair step increasing trial of DSMO to glycerol.

13.7 AMIDES

Amides have proven to be a mostly beneficial CPA, having been shown to decrease damaging results compared to those obtained when glycerol is solely used as the CPO. With stallions being sorted into different freezing classes, poor freezers have required substantial work. Amides have increased the freezing potential of this class while subsequently decreasing the overall damaging results induced from glycerol. While glycerol is still the main CPA used for stallion sperm, the addition of amides, in part due to their lower viscosity and molecular weight, may decrease sperm cell damage. DMF has been shown to enhance post-thaw motility, preservation cellular membranes which may effectively enhancing semen freezing potential. With lower molecular weights, both DMF and MF are able to permeate stallion sperm, more efficiently than glycerol, which has resulted in reduced swelling during equilibration in amide-containing diluents and not as toxic as glycerol. However, DMF and MF seem to be the only amides with possible cryogenic effects. Studies have shown that other amides have detrimental effects on semen not being cryoprotective.

As previously discussed, stallion sperm is highly individualistic, because of this; research into additional CPA's that would help to preserve frozen semen has flourished. The discovery of MF and DMF as agents has been more than beneficial to the industry and spurred investigation of other alternative agents. Reductions of freezing and thawing damage, improving membrane integrity and increasing progressive motility have been the goal of equine cryobiology researchers over the last 30years. During that time, reducing damage due to freezing and thawing has been the focus of most investigating alternative CPA's. Recently, work with the addition of liposomes, which induce fusion to the sperm plasma membranes, as well as the reversible binding of exogenous phospholipids, have both shown to protect sperm from damage. Cholesterol and methyl-β cyclodetrin[31] have been shown to reduce membrane transition temperatures, resulting in reduced cryoinjury, maintenance of the cellular membranes and improve post-thaw motility. Like most potential CPA, the use of a lipid based CPO has been demonstrated to have both positive and negative effects on equine semen.

13.8 LIPIDS

Previous studies have demonstrated CP can lead to loss of from the membrane leading to peroxidation and continuing on to form reactive oxidative species.[32] Lipid bases are multifaceted since they have been linked to both oxidation of, as well as the protection of lipid bilayer infusions. The addition of a lipid based CPO may destabilize the sperm membrane due to the formation of ROS and recruitment of lipids from the membrane leading to lipid rearrangement within the membrane itself causing additional oxidation to occur. Increased peroxidation in turn might affect both motility and acrosomal activity. Sperm are prone to cold shock damage due to osmotic stress and relative temperatures which in turn may lead to underlying damage to the integrity of membrane. Further studies are need to determine the exact role lipids play in protecting spermatozoa during freeze-thaw is unclear. Therefore if lipids are to be added as a cryoprotective agent to produce a more saturated CPO for semen preservation, there are a few other issues which must address. Numerous studies have shown that ROS play a significant role in male infertility. Further, cold shock damage has been directly linked to lipid phase transitions that cause the sperm membrane to become leaky, thereby compromising membrane integrity. However, ROS been shown a double-edged sword. While their detrimental effects are well documented, at low levels they are involved in the normal physiological functions of sperm including capacitation, acrosome reaction, and binding to the Zona pellucida at physiological concentrations.

13.9 OPTIMIZING FORMULAS

While the usage of amino acids with stallion sperm has not been studied extensively, the few studies done today suggest they may be an important addition to extender formulations. Koskinen et al.[36] demonstrated the addition of betaine, as a stallion CPA, which stimulated increased post-thaw motility.[36] Initial testing from Sanchez-Partida et al. working with frozen ram sperm demonstrated low concentrations of proline, glycine and betaine could be used to improve post-thaw motility as well.[37] Trimeche et al. also showed that low concentrations of proline to be beneficial in enhancing the motility parameters of stallion sperm. Glutamine has been helpful when combined with glycerol for human sperm post-thaw motility and viability, and at low concentrations, it has worked effectively in stallion semen. Conversely, high concentrations of betaine, glutamine, histidine and proline were demonstrated to cause significant dropped in sample motility. As mentioned above, work has been done with other amides as well. However, unlike the beneficial effects described for MF and DMF, acetamide, and formamide both appear to be toxic to stallion semen, and have poor cryoprotective properties which make them unsuitable as a CPA.

13.10 MEMBRANE ISSUES

Baird's Tapir are evolutionarily related to equids and rhinoceros. Tapir's semen osmolality has proven similar to that of the domestic horse, Prezwalskis horse, and the rhinoceros.[41] However, the average pH of the samples being lower than the three aforementioned species, the difference can be attributed to accessory gland contributions. Due to the shared evolutionary relationship between these species, the industry knowledge that has been acquired for stallions may help to determine appropriate CP techniques and CPA that may be applicable for the other equid species. With stallions, it has been proven that the addition of cholesterol helps to increase the spermatozoa permeability to CPO thereby increasing the osmotic tolerance, and improving the sperm cryosurvival rates. Given the semen osmolality similarities it has been suggested that cholesterol be included, to help facilitate better Tapir semen preservation.

One particular challenge for the Tapir, as with any non-domesticated specie, is the collection of the sample. While domesticated stallions are able to be collected via an artificial vagina, this is an unrealistic approach to nondomestic species, as Tapirs would be more at risk to injury.

Prezwalskis' have not been cryobiologically studied, and therefore currently rely on research information gather from the domestic horse, especially concerning sperm cryosensitivity.[42] It is a well-established fact that less than 20% of domestic stallions produce sperm that are capable meaningful post-thaw survival, mainly due to the variations in individual CP capacities. This appears to be the case with the Prezwalskis as well. As in any species, there is the challenge of minimizing toxic CPO impacts are vital. However, there is evidence that amides will help to mitigate toxic impact of these compounds. Current research has suggested that Prezwalskis spermatozoa are tolerant of cryoagents, cryodilutents, and the processing used in the domestic horse industry. These findings give hope for the potential of CP of a species that is facing extinction.

13.11 CRYONJURY

Mazurs two factor hypothesis on freezing injury, helps to categorize and explain the freezing responses from different cell types. The osmotic behavior of cells is widely understood, respectively with each species and cell type, having unique boundaries. However, the increased variation between stallions compared to other species, make this less predictable. Recently, it has been shown that rapid cooling of human and stallion sperm infers a loss of viability, but more interestingly suggested that intracellular ice may not be the culprit.[44] Demonstrating how speeding up the cooling rates, Morris et al. would reduce the ice crystallization damage by "solution effects." They also suggested that those same higher cooling rates are found in glycerol solutions. Given what we know about stallion sperm, this relationship appears counterintuitive, as the majority of glycerol based CPO's have been shown to have a more deleterious effect on sperm cells. Morris also suggested that post-thaw semen quality might be just as dependent on semen concentration as well as any single CPA of the additive.

Finally, in addition to the biochemical and physiological issues above, both the methodologies used for collection as well as the mechanics preparing sperm for freezing may result in significant cell loss. While many techniques are more than suitable for producing a fertile sample, the loss of semen is inevitable and can be classified into the following: loss during receptacle transfer, loss in centrifuge tubes, loss due to air exposure, with cautionary techniques used, there is still loss involved, most of which can be attributed to extended air exposure. Stallion sperm can use both aerobic and anaerobic pathways and with fluxing temperature and air exposure, the concept of motility conservation minus air exposure results in the decline of energy stores via glycolysis and glycogen recruitment.

A basic understanding of the architecture of the sperm membrane is crucial to understand how cryoinjury occurs to cells. Nowhere is this more true and with more impact on fertility than damage to the acrosomal membrane. Membrane composition and fluidity of the individual lipid bilayer is highly dependent on the dietary intake. The intercalation of CPO or other compounds affect membrane fluidity, cause changes to the cytoplasmic viscosity, ultimately affecting the cell's metabolic capacity. Concurrently, when cells are introduced to low temperatures that they would not normally physiologically encounter, the membrane alters its mechanism of lipid packing, which modifies enzymes within the membrane and the kinetic properties of the cells. All of these factors lead to the imminent potential of cryoinjury, including: cold shock, freezing damage or thawing damage.

13.12 APOPTOSIS

Apoptosis can occur within all cells, resulting in programmed cell death. The physiological process of programmed cell death which affects single cells and induces morphological and biochemical changes which lead to cell death and acts as a homeostatic function within the body. It has been shown to occur within spermatogenesis as a homeostatic event, to help balance the new and old cells. Since apoptosis is required to allow the normal development of germ cells, spermatogenic apoptosis helps to maintain the balance between germ and somatic cells, while also removing the defective germ cells. However if this process is interrupted it could lead to increased quantities of ejaculates spermatozoa displaying apoptotic like changes and result in decreased fertility. With a two-pathway option for apoptotic initiation, the intrinsic is due to pre-apoptotic signals that lead to the activation of caspases, and extrinsically death receptor pathway receptors allow for ligand binding to occur at the plasma membrane again leading to activation of caspases. The current two theory methodology for apoptosis include abortive apoptosis which is the marking of defective germ cells during spermatogenesis, but instead of apoptosis occurring, they are able to escape the testes. The second theory is mature ejaculated spermatozoa are undergoing apoptosis or an apoptosis like process; initially this was thought to have not occurred, but recent studies have shown that ejaculated sperm are capable of triggering caspase activation.

Spermatozoa are exposed to a variety of physical and chemical stresses during CP, changing the lipid composition of the plasma membrane, head size as well as resulting in DNA damage[49] and increased plasma membrane lipid disorder allowing the supposition that apoptotic like changes may be induced in equine sperm CP.

A portion of the cell loss that occurs during CP as cells already programmed to die are included in the freezing process and may reduce the number of viable cells in an AI dosage. Moreover some of the more subtle damage that is caused to sperm cells via CP may help to induce this programmed cell death, and therefore lower viability numbers transferred and/or reduced life span of those cells when in the female reproductive tract. The apoptotic phenomena of cryopreserved stallion's sperm is attributed to oxidative stress, phase transitions of the plasma membranes, cryocapacitation, as well as the premature activation of the pathway due to subtle damages. Unfortunately, without extensive testing, there is no easy way to determine a cell that has begun the apoptotic process. These defective cells are programmed for removal, but unfortunately with only one pathway out, the expulsion of dead cells occurs consistently within the ejaculate.

A cause of apoptosis normally overlooked during semen processing is the presence of microbes in the semen sample.[19] Results from a more recent study has shown that stallions ejaculate is more in line with that of humans due to the bacteria which induce sperm apoptosis[51] and necrosis;[52] with the microbial flora playing a critical role in the sublethal apoptotic damage that stallion spermatozoa experience during CP and cooled storage.

13.13 REACTIVE OXYGEN SPECIES

A recent set of studies looked the activity of proteins, apoptosis and ROS, the proteins involved in the activation of apoptosis and the inductor protein involved in the activation of the mitochondrial pathway of apoptosis-have been found in fresh, frozen and thawed equine spermatozoa.[54,] Together these studies support the idea that ejaculated spermatozoa can trigger activation the nuclear matrix potentially leading to cleavage of the entire sperm DNA into small fragments. There is still controversy about the apoptotic markers that have been found in equine semen subpopulations and if this information is actually a significant, subsequent information collected post CP would need to be done for analysis for equine semen.

Further, depending on training of individuals involved, counts may include no sperm cells such as residual bodies. Residual bodies are made from cytoplasmic portions of elongated spermatids,[50] and are subsequently shed with viable sperm cells into the seminiferous tubules, and therefore into the ejaculate.

Osmotic shock (OS) has long been associated with and a major factor in sperm damage during cryopreservation; and while this statement still holds true, newer research demonstrates it is just one potential problem. The influx of hypertonic concentrations while freezing and the hypotonic concentrations when thawing have been shown to induce OS which has been shown to be detrimental to the integrity of sperm cells. Somatic cells have been well documented to show that OS is responsible for apoptosis, cell cycle arrest, DNA damage, oxidative stress as well as a variety of other actions.

This is especially true in stallions, as spermatozoa have a very limited osmotic threshold[57] which ultimately results in uncontrollable shrinking and swelling of the sperm head causing damage to the semen. Studies have shown that stallion sperm damaged during flash freezing and morphologically abnormal sperm generate greater amounts of ROS. While the fluidity of the plasmalemma is able to tolerate and adjust to these changes without penalty, OS may lead to a loss in viability, poor motility, and/or a decrease in the mitochondrial membrane potential.

Peroxidation of plasma membrane lipids (lipid peroxidation, LPO) has been proposed to be a major factor involved in sub-lethal cryodamage of sperm in many species, including horses. Two pathways may result in the formation of LPO's; the enzymatic membrane system using NAD(P)H as a substrate and the mitochondrial electron transport chain. The main source of oxidative stress for spermatozoa is the mitochondria. ROS production is increased in sperm mitochondria due to freezing and thawing, while an osmotic mechanism may increase mitochondrial membrane permeability, thus activating apoptosis. In fact, oxidative stress is a well-documented inductor of apoptosis.[58] The concept of relative osmotic stress to the hyper and hypotonic environments has been shown to define the range, which may represent the "osmotic tolerance limit." Once these limits are surpassed, they cause irreversible damage to the cell, preventing the spermatozoa from recovering its initial motility when returned to isosmolality environment. Pommer et al. suggested this hypertonic limit for motility was reached at 450mOsm/kg while Garcia et al. demonstrated a hypertonic effect at 1500mOsm/kg, which prevented stallion spermatozoa from recovering their initial volume once osmotic balance was restored.

13.14 FUTURE OF SEMEN CRYOPRESERVATION

As should be apparent from the forgoing material, CP of equine semen is desired by the industry as a means of long-term preservation and storage of superior genetics. While the vast majority of the research has focused on CPO's, there remains a need for a simpler device that is able to provide the same quality results, which we are currently obtaining from the programmable freezers. Equine CP, has be something which has been more than problematic for the industry, and just within the past ten years we have broken through to new methods which are allowing us to achieve the idea of a superior yet simple device. Programmable freezers using electricity have been the detriment to stallions, and the poor post thaw recovery rates generated from vertical mist have pushed the industry forward. The reduced quality of semen post-thaw is a clear response to the sub-optimal cryopreservation protocols that are in use, as the majority of cellular damage has been reported to occur between in the initial freezing stages. Ideally an optimal freezing rate must be slow enough to prevent intracellular ice formation, but fast enough to avoid cryoinjury. The necessity for a simpler device has been acknowledged and the equine reproductive industry has begun to explore alternative options. With sperm being susceptible to rapid cold shock injuries especially during the initial process and leading to membrane damage, the goal of this study was to slowly yet effectively control and decrease the temperature.

RELATED TERMINOLOGY

Albumen Firmness: Quality description of the albumen (egg white) of an egg. Albumen is judged on the basis of clarity and firmness or thickness. A clear albumen is defined as being free from discolorations or from any foreign bodies.

Animal Model: Mathematical approach to determine the genetic and environmental factors which may affect animal performances. This system allows an accurate prediction of the breeding values of future reproducers. The Animal Model simultaneously evaluates dams (♀) and sires (♂) using all their ancestor relationships. This means that every animal known in a given pedigree is used to evaluate both the dam and sire. This increases the accuracy of evaluation and should be a major step in breeder acceptance of the new evaluation system.

APHA:– Animal and Plant Health Agency: governing body tasked with protecting the health and welfare of animals.

Artificial Fertilisation: The bringing together of semen and eggs under laboratory conditions.

Artificial Insemination: Collecting semen from a male and bringing this into the genital tract of a female.

Atresia ani: Hereditary genetic defect: animals are born without anus.

AV:–Artificial Vagina: tool used to collect semen from a bull and ram.

Balanced Breeding: Breeding for a combination of characteristics, concerning animal biology, animal health, efficiency, environment, animal welfare and economy.

BCS:– Body Conditioning Score: numeric score to estimate body energy reserves in the cow

Best Linear Unbiased Prediction (BLUP): A statistical method, that gives the estimation of Breeding Values. This is a rating or breeding quality number and is a prediction of the breeding potential of the individual animal and how likely it is that that animal will improve (or not improve) its offspring. BLUP calculations are used to predict the genetic make-up of an animal for all kinds of traits. With BLUP it is possible to track and predict the different inherited traits through complicated mathematical and statistical calculations.

Biotechnology: Technology that utilises biology to reap benefits for the herd. Often this involves creating or modifying DNA to select optimum genetic traits.

Bovine Leukocyte Adhesion Deficiency (BLAD): is a hereditary genetic disease (detected in the Holstein breed), an adhesion deficiency of bovine leukocytes to antigens, which shows in calves as not being able to recover after an illness. A DNA-test is available to detect animals that are carriers of the defect allele.

Bovine Spongiform Encephalopathy (BSE): sometimes known as "mad cow" disease, is a prion disease of cattle first identified in 1986. BSE occurs in adult animals in both sexes, typically in four and five year olds. It is a neurological disease involving pronounced changes in mental state, abnormalities of posture and movement and of sensation. The clinical disease usually lasts for several weeks. Only a small proportion of affected cattle show what would be considered typical "mad cow" signs. Possibly, when humans eat meat from an infected animal, they develop a similar disease. Creutzfeldt-Jacob Disease (CJD) is a rare and fatal neurodegenerative disease of unknown cause.

Breeding Organisation (BO): Organisation involved in the breeding of farm animals.

Breeding value: The estimated genetic value of an individual. The part of an individual's genotypic value that is due to independent and therefore transmittable gene effects.

Broiler: A type of chicken bred for meat production.

Calving Rate: This is the total number of services received by a group of cows which result in calving as a percentage of the total number of services.

Calving: The birth of one or more calves more than 270 days following an effective service.

Cervix:- Neck like structure, opening towards the uterus.

Challenge Test: Tests designed to identify differences between individuals, families, lines or strain crosses in their ability to cope with diseases or stress factors likely to be encountered in practice. Results from challenge tests are used to select relatives for improved resistance. In case of transmittable diseases, test farms are operated with maximal bio-security.

CIDR:– Controlled Internal Drug Release: device which releases progesterone to allow control of a cow's oestrus cycle .

Cloning (Somatic): Producing offspring with the same genetic information, e.g. embryonic cloning, identical twins.

Complex Vertebral Malformation (CVM): Genetic defect in cattle associated with the disorder range from earlier embryonic death to late term stillborn calves with neck and leg deformities. A DNA-test is available to detect animals that are carrier of the defect allele.

Conception:- The onset of pregnancy.

Congenital Defects: Defects present at birth.

Cryopreservation: Preservation by means of freezing, e.g. semen, embryos.

Cryptorchism: Hereditary genetic disease (genetic defect) in which testicles are not descended.

Embryo Transfer: Recovering embryos from a donor animal and transferring these embryos to a recipient animal.

Cull Cow: A cow that is removed from the herd.

Dairy Nutritionist: Expert animal health consultants who advise on the nutritional needs of cows. They help recommend the best diets for maximising the fertility of each cow.

Dam: The mother of a calf.

Date of Conception: The date of the effective service.

Date of Service: The date of the first natural mating or artificial insemination.

Degenerate Embryo:- A fertilised embryo that is dead or dying embryo and is deemed unsuitable for embryo transfer or freezing.

DFR:- Dominant Follicle Reduction: procedure implemented during the stimulation process whereby a needle is used to remove the biggest follicles which can have an inhibitory effect on other follicles

Ejaculation:- The release of semen through the penis during orgasm.

Embryo Loss: When a developing calf does not survive during the first 42 days of pregnancy.

Embryo:- Having to do with an early stage in the development of a plant or an animal. In vertebrate animals, this stage lasts from shortly after fertilization until all major body parts appear. In particular, in humans, this stage lasts from about 2 weeks after fertilization until the end of the seventh or eighth week of pregnancy.

Endometrium:- This is the mucous membrane comprising the inner layer of the utrine wall.

Fallopian tubes:- Structures between the ovaries and the uterus through which the egg travels to the uterus.

Farm Animal Breeding: Strategies applied by specialized farmers to increase desirable traits selecting the appropriate animals as ancestors of the new generations.

Fertilization:- Process of conception in which the sperm penetrates the egg (ovum).

Foetal loss: When a foetus dies between 43 and 151 days of pregnancy.

Foetus: The developing calf from day 43 to birth.

Follicle:- fluid filled cavity in the ovary containing one oocyte. An ovary contains multiple follicles are any given stage of the oestrus cycle.

FSH:- Follicle Stimulating Hormone: hormone given to cows to stimulate production of many oocytes

Gametes:- Sperm or ovum (egg); the cells of reproduction.

Genetically modified organism (GMO): When a copy of a gene is made from one organism and then used in another organism. This helps improve plants or other organism by allowing the selection of specific beneficial genes.

Genome Wide Selection (Genomic Selection): Use of total breeding values for juvenile animals, predicted from a large number of estimated marker haplotype effects across the whole genome. Single Nucleotide Polymorphisms (SNPs) are used as high-density markers in genome wide selection.

Genetic Diversity: High variety of alleles of genes within a population.

Haugh Units: A measure of the firmness of albumen in the eggs, correcting albumen height for variable egg weight (layer chicken).

Genotype: The genetic constitution of an animal.

Gestation Period: The number of days between conception and birth.

GMO Feed: A feed that has had ingredients altered or modified by genetic engineering.

Heat Oestrus – Stage in the oestrus cycle where the oocyte is released from the ovary; occurs every 18 to 24 days

Heifer: A mature female cow that is yet to give birth.

Hermaphrodism: Biological mode of reproduction in which an individual presents alternatively or simultaneously male and female territory in its gonad.

IMF: Intramuscular fat or marbling of muscle meat.

In Vitro Embryo Production: The production of embryos outside an animals' body using sperm and unfertilised eggs.

Inbreeding: genes that two animals have in common due to common anchestors. Inbreeding can be used to increase genetic variation between families in order to increase response to selection. In commercial breeding programmes, inbreeding is seldom used. Loss of genetic diversity due to inbreeding depends on effective population size and selection intensity.

In-Calf Heifer: A heifer that has been confirmed to be in calf.

Infertility:- The inability to produce children.

Interbull: International breeding value estimation in dairy cattle. Interbull is a non-profit organisation, responsible for the standardisation of international genetic evaluations for cattle. In practice this means, that a French farmer may use semen from a South American bull with known breeding value for French conditions, because the international breeding value is comparable globally. There is an extensive international trade of bull semen, globally.

Inter-Service Interval: The amount of days between the last service of a cow to the next, during the same lactation.

Intrauterine - Within the cavity of the uterus.

IVF (In vitro fertilization):- The process by which the egg is fertilized outside the body, then transferred

IVP:– In Vitro Production: entire process including oocyte collection and maturation (TVR/OPU), IVF, and embryo culture to produce embryos within a specialised laboratory

Layer: A type of chicken bred for efficient egg production.

Leucosis: A malignant disease of the lymphatic system in chickens, caused by a virus. Marker assisted selection (MAS): Selection using genomic markers. The idea behind marker assisted selection is that there may be genes with significant effects that may be targeted specifically in selection. Some traits are controlled by single genes (e.g. hair colour) but most traits of economic importance are quantitative traits that most likely are controlled by a fairly large number of genes. However, some of these genes might have a larger effect.

Maiden Heifer: A heifer that has not had a service.

Mass Selection: A form of selection in which only individuals with phenotypic values greater or less than a threshold level are used for breeding. It involves no use of family information. (Compare with pedigree selection).

Mastitis: Mammary gland or udder inflammation caused by various species of bacteria

MF: Mule Foot is a genetic defect in cattle expressed as fused hoofs. A marker-test is available to detect animals that are carriers of the defect allele.

Metritis – Inflammation of the wall of the uterus

MOET – Multiple Ovulation and Embryo Transfer, also known as flushing

Monofactorial Genetic Effects: One gene being responsible for a certain genetic effect, e.g. halothane gene, BLAD, CVM.

Monosex population: production of population of animals of only one phenotypic sex by gamete management (sperm sexing, gynogenesis, sex inversion) or by the control of environmental factors as grading or for example in fish by the application of hot or cold temperature during the sexual differentiation period.

Muscle Hypertrophy: Extreme growth of skeletal muscle as in some breeds of cattle, sheep, pigs (double muscling).

Mycoplasma: Pathogenic bacteria causing many diseases of humans, plants and animals. Due to their specific structure they have low sensitivity to the effect of antibiotics.

N and P Emission: All animals require Nitrogen and Phosphorus in their feed and when they produce manure it will contain some N and P. This is brought into the environment, e.g. grassland or arable land. If the growth period and need of the crop are not consistent with the amount of N (Nitrogen) or P (Phosphorus) brought on the land, N and P may leak into the air, lakes, rivers or ground water. Animals digesting their feed efficiently will pollute the environment less.

Oestrus Cycle Length: Duration of time from the start of the oestrus cycle to the beginning of the next. The start of the first oestrus is counted as Day 0.

Oestrus Cycle: The regular advent of oestrus / coming into heat, this comes with a change in the genitals and reproductive hormones.

Oestrus Induction: Hormonal stimulation of oestrus at desired moment to ensure a better control and care of reproducers and offspring.

Oocyte – unfertilised egg produced by cows. Collected and fertilised by semen to produce an embryo.

OPU – Ovum Pick Up: stage in IVP whereby oocytes are collected from the multiple follicles on an ovary.

Osteoporosis: Osteoporosis is a disease in which bones become fragile and more likely to break.

Polledness: An animal born without the potential to grow horns.

Pregnancy - Growth of an embryo/fetus in the uterus.

Premature Calving: This term refers to the birth of one or more calves between 152 and 270 days after an effective service. The calf must survive for 24 hours or more.

Progesterone/Prostaglandin – Naturally occurring hormones which allow control of the oestrus cycle when applied externally.

Replacement Rate: The number of cows or heifers that are required to replace the cows that have left the herd during a period (usually 12 months) as a percentage of the total average herd size.

Salmonella: Salmonella is a bacterium. There is a widespread occurrence in animals, especially in poultry and swine. Environmental sources of the organism include water, soil, insects, factory surfaces, kitchen surfaces, animal faeces, raw meats, raw poultry, and raw seafoods. Humans infected with Salmonella bacteria can get nausea, abdominal cramps, diarrhea, fever, headache or vomit.

Somatic Cell Count: The somatic cell count (SCC) is commonly used as a measure of milk quality. Somatic cells are simply animal body cells present at low levels in normal milk. High levels of these cells in milk indicate abnormal, reduced-quality milk that is caused by an intramammary bacterial infection (mastitis).

Semen - Thick, whitish fluid containing sperms that is discharged through the penis during ejaculation.

Served Heifer: A heifer that has been served, or has transferred an embryo, but is yet to be confirmed to be in calf.

Service: One or more natural or artificial inseminations during a period of oestrus.

Sperm Sexing: Separation of male and female spermatozoa. After the sexing procedure, the semen can be used to produce predominantly male or female offspring.

Sperm - Male reproductive cells produced by the testes and transported in the semen; spermatozoa.

Urethra - The tube through which urine leaves the body. It empties urine from the bladder.

Vagina - The passage (birth canal) connecting the female external genitalia with the uterus.

Vasectomy - An operation to cut or tie off the two tubes that carry sperm out of the testicles.

Sponge – Synchronisation of oestrus and ovulation in sheep.

Stillborn Calf: A calf that has been birthed dead or found dead after an unobserved calving.

Stimulation/Super Ovulation – Process of injecting reproductive hormones to improve oocyte quality or number by promoting follicle growth.

Sudden Death Syndrome: Birds (broiler chickens) which have died suddenly are found on their backs with no other obvious pathology. The cause is probably metabolic. It can be induced by lactic acidosis and about 70% of birds affected are males.

Sustainability: Sustainability in farm animal breeding and reproduction means the extent to which animal breeding and reproduction, as managed by professional organisations, contribute to maintenance and good care of animal genetic resources for present and future generations (www.sefabar.org).

Traceability: Organisation of a production process in such a way that all the steps can be 'traced'. E.g. when a piece of meat is bought in a supermarket, it should be possible to 'trace' back to the farm where it was produced, and to the parents of the animal.

Triploidy: biological mechanism happening in which an individual developed with 3 sets of chromosomes (i.e.: 2 of its mothers and 1 from his father) instead of 2 in diploids (1 from each of its parents).

TVR – Trans Vaginal Recovery: process by which OPU is carried out in cows.

UFO – Unfertilised Embryo.

Weaning: Accustom animals to do without the mother's milk (mammals) or leaving prey (fish).

Yolk/Albumen Ratio: Amount of yolk compared to amount of albumen in an egg. It can be used as a measure of egg quality in layer breeding programmes.

Zoonotic Disease: Disease that can be transmitted from animals to humans.

Zoonotic Risk: Risk that an animal disease will be transmitted to humans.

REFERENCES

Abecia, J. A., F. Forcada, and A. Gonzalez-Bulnes. 2012. Hormonal control of reproduction in small ruminants. Animal Reproduction Science 130: 173-179.

Aitkin ID (1991) Enzootic (Chlamydial) abortion in Diseases of sheep ed. WB Martin and ID Aitken 2nd ed Blackwell Scientific Publications pp 43-49.

Ak K, Ak S, Gurel A, Hasoksuz M, Baran A, Ozturkler Y, Ileri IK, Minbay A (1995) Experimental studies on the effects of Mycoplasma agalactia on the spermatozoa and genital organs of rams Pendik Veterinar Mikrobiyoloji Dergisis 26: 139-155.

Al Yacoub, A. N., M. Gauly, and W. Holtz. 2010. Open pulled straw vitrification of goat embryos at various stages of development. Theriogenology 73: 1018-1023.

Al Yacoub, A. N., M. Gauly, B. Sohnrey, and W. Holtz. 2011. Fixed-time deep uterine insemination in PGF2alpha-synchronized goats. Theriogenology 76: 1730-1735.

Althouse GC, Wilson ME, Kuster C, et al. Characterization of lower temperature storage limitations of fresh-extended porcine semen. Theriogenology. 1998;50(4):535–543.

Alton GG (1984) The epidemiology of Brucella melitensis infection in sheep and goats in Brucella melitensis. Current topics in veterinary medicine and animal science vol. 32 ed. JM Verger and M Plommet pp.187-196.

Alvarenga MA, Papa FO, Landim-Alvarenga FC, et al. Amides as cryoprotectants for freezing stallion semen: A review. Animal Reproduction Science. 2005;89(1-4):105–113.

Amiridis, G. S., and S. Cseh. 2012. Assisted reproductive technologies in the reproductive management of small ruminants. Animal Reproduction Science 130: 152-161.

Anon (1981) Disease control in semen and embryos – report of the expert consultation on animal disease control in international movement of semen and embryos, Food and Agriculture Organization of the United nations Rome 1981.

Appleyard WT, Aitken ID, Anderson IE (1985) Attempted venereal transmission of Chlamydia psittaci in sheep. Vet Rec 116:535-8.

Aurich JE. Artificial insemination in horses-more than a century of practice and research. Journal of Equine Veterinary Science. 2012;32(8):458–463.

Awda BJ, Mackenzie-Bell M, Buhr MM. Reactive oxygen species and boar sperm function. Biol Reprod. 2009;81(3):553–561.

Bai C, Wang X, Lu G, et al. Cooling rate optimization for zebra fish sperm cryopreservation using a cryomicroscope coupled with SYBR14/PI dual staining. Cryobiology. 2013;67(2):117–123.

Bai J, Bishop JV, Carlson JO, DeMartini JC (1999) Sequence comparison of JSRV with endogenous proviruses: envelope genotypes and a novel ORF with similarity to a G-protein-coupled receptor Virology 258:333-43

Bailey JL, Blodeau JF, Cormier N. Semen Cryopreservation in Domestic Animals: A Damaging and Capacitating Phenomenon Minireview. Journal of Andrology. 2000;21(1):1–7.

Ball BA, Vo A. Osmotic tolerance of equine spermatozoa and the effects of soluble cryoprotectants on equine sperm motility, viability, and mitochondrial membrane potential. J Androl. 2001; 22(6):1061–1069.

Bane A (1981) Diseases of sheep and goats in relation to artificial insemination with frozen semen in Disease control in semen and embryos – report of the expert consultation on animal disease control in international movement of semen and embryos, Food and Agriculture Organization of the United nations Rome 1981

Banks KL, Adams DS, McGuire TC, Carlson J (1983) Experimental infection of sheep by caprine-arthritis encephalitis virus and goats by progressive ovine pneumonia virus Am J Vet Res 44: 2307-11

Benson JD, Woods EJ, Walters EM, et al. The cryobiology of spermatozoa. Theriogenology. 2012;78(8):1682-1699.

Bercovich Z, Guler L, Baysal T, Schreuder BEC, van Zijderveld FG (1998) Evaluation of the currently used diagnostic procedures for the detection of Brucella melitensis in sheep. Small Ruminant Research 31: 1-6.

Bergonier D, Berthelot X, Poumarat F (1997) Contagious agalactia of small ruminants: current knowledge concerning epidemiology, diagnosis and control. Rev Sci Tech 16:848-73

Blasco JM, Garin-Bastuji B, Marin CM, Gerbier G, Fanlo J, Jimenez de Bagues MP, Cau C (1994) Efficacy of different Rose Bengal and complement fixation antigens for the diagnosis of Brucella melitensis infection in sheep and goats. Vet Rec 134: 415-420.

Blottner S, Warnke C, Tuchscherer A, et al. Morphological and functional changes of stallion spermatozoa after cryopreservation during breeding and non-breeding season. Animal Reproduction Science. 2001;65(1–2):75-88.

Bodin, L., P. V. Drion, B. Remy, G. Brice, Y. Cognie, and J. F. Beckers. 1997. Anti-PMSG antibody levels in sheep subjected annually to oestrus synchronisation. Reprod Nutr Dev 37: 651-660.

Bolske G, Johansson KE, Heinonen R, Panvuga PA, Twinamasiko E (1995) Contagious caprine pleuropneumonia in Uganda and isolation of Mycoplasma capricolum subspecies capripneumoniae from sheep and goats. Vet Rec 137: 594

Boumedine KS, Rodolakis A (1998) AFLP allows the identification of genomic markers of ruminant Chlamydia psittaci strains useful for typing and epidemiological studies. Res Microbiol 149:735-44

Bowdridge, E. C., W. B. Knox, C. S. Whisnant, and C. E. Farin. 2013. NCSynch: A novel, progestagen-free protocol for ovulation synchronization and timed artificial insemination in goats. Small Ruminant Research 110: 42-45.

Bowen JM. Artificial insemination in the horse. Equine Veterinary Journal. 1969;1(3):98–110.

Brodie SJ, de la Concha-Bermajillo, Koenig G, Snowder GD, DeMartini JC (1994) Maternal factors associated with prenatal transmission of ovine lentivirus. J Infect Dis 169;653-657

Broekhuijse, M. L., H. Feitsma, and B. M. Gadella. 2012. Artificial insemination in pigs: predicting male fertility. The Veterinary quarterly 32: 151-157.

Brown AS, Amos ML, Lavin MF, Girjes AA, Timms P, Woolcock JB (1988) Isolation and typing of a strain of Chlamydia psittaci from Angora goats Aust Vet J 65: 288-289

Buonavoglia D, Fasanella A, Greco G, Pratelli A (1999) A study of an experimental infection of sheep with Mycoplasma agalactiae. New Microbiol 22:27-30

Burgess GW, Spencer TL, Norris MJ (1985) Experimental infection of goats with Brucella ovis. Aust Vet J 62: 262-264

Carey N and Dalziel RG (1993) The biology of maedi-visna- an overview. Br Vet J 149: 437-453

Carn VM, Timms CP, Chand P, Black DN, Kitching RP (1994) Protection of goats against capripox using a subunit vaccine. Vet Rec 135: 434-436

Castro RS, Greenland T, Leite RC, Gouveia A, Mornex JF, Cordier G (1999) Conserved sequence motifs involving the tat reading frame of Brazilian caprine lentiviruses indicate affiliations to both caprine arthritis-encephalitis virus and visna-maedi virus.J Gen Virol 80:1583-9

Cerri D, Nuvoloni R, Ebani V, Pedrini A, Mani P, Andreani E, Farina R (1996) Leptospira interrogans serovar hardjo in the kidneys and genital tracts of naturally infected sheep. New Microbiol 19:175-8

Chan R, Hardiman RP (1993) Endocarditis caused by Brucella melitensis. Med J Aust 158:631-2

Chand P, Kitching RP and Black DN (1994) Western blot analysis of virus-specific antibody responses to capripox and contagious pustular dermatitis infections in sheep. Epid Infect 113: 377-385

Chemineau P, Procureur R, Cognie Y, Lefevre PC, Locatelli A, Chupin D (1986) Production, freezing and transfer of embryos from a bluetongue-infected goat herd without bluetongue transmission. Theriogenology 26: 279-290

Chen SS and Wrathall AE (1989) The importance of the zona pellucida for disease control in livestock by embryo transfer. Brit Vet J 145: 129-140

Chlamydia psittaci strains infecting koalas (Phascolarctos cinereus). Vet Microbiol 37:65-83

Collins DM, Gabric DM, and de Lisle GW (1990) Identification of two groups of M paratuberculosis strains by restriction endonuclease analysis and DNA hybridization J Clin Microbiol 28: 1591-1596.

Constable PD, Meier WA, Foley GL, Morin D, Cutlip RC, Zachary JF (1996) Visna-like disease in a ram with chronic demyelinating encephalomyelitis. JAVMA 208: 117-120

Contreras A, Corrales JC, Sanchez A, Aduriz JJ, Gonzalez L, Marco J (1998) Caprine arthritis- encephalitis in an indigenous Spanish breed of dairy goat.Vet Rec 142:140-2

Cottew GS and Yeats FR (1982) Mycoplasmas and mites in the ears of clinically normal goats. Aust Vet J 59: 77-81

Crabo BG. Physiological aspects of stallion semen cryopreservation. Proceedings of the Annual Convention - American Association of Equine Practitioners. 2001;47:291–295.

Cross RF, Smith CK, Moorhead PD (1975) Vertical transmission of progressive pneumonia (maedi) in sheep. Am J Veter Res 36:465-468.

Cseh, S., V. Faigl, and G. S. Amiridis. 2012. Semen processing and artificial insemination in health management of small ruminants. Animal Reproduction Science 130: 187-192.

Curry MR. Cryopreservation of semen from domestic livestock. Reviews of Reproduction. 2000;5(1):46–52.

Cutlip RC (1992) Seroprevalence of ovine progressive pneumonia virus in sheep in the United States as assessed by analyses of voluntarily submitted samples. Am J Vet Res 53: 976-9.

Cutlip RC, Lehmkuhl HD, Brogden KA, Sacks JM (1986) Breed susceptibility to ovine progressive pneumonia (maedi/visna) virus. Vet Microbiol 12: 283-8

Cutlip RC, Lehmkuhl HD, Jackson TA (1981) Intrauterine transmission of ovine progressive pneumonia virus Am J Vet Res 42:1795-1797

Cutlip RC, Lehmkuhl HD, Schmerr MJ, Brogden KA (1988) Ovine progressive pneumonia (maedi-visna) in sheep. Vet Microbiol 17: 237-50

Cutlip RC, Young S (1982) Sheep pulmonary adenomatosis (Jaagsiekte) in the United States Am J Vet Res 43: 2108-2113

Davidson JN, Hirsh DC (1980) Leptospirosis in lambs. J Am Vet Med Assoc 176:124 Davies FG (1997) Tick virus diseases of sheep and goats Parasitologia. 39: 91-4

De Boer GF, Terpestra C, Hendrinks J ,Houwers DJ (1979) Studies in epidemiology of maedi-visna in sheep. Res Vet Sc 26: 202-208

De la Concha-Bermejillo A, Magnus-Corral S, Brodie SJ, DeMartini JC (1996) Venereal shedding of ovine lentivirus in infected rams. AVJR 57: 684-688

Dedieu L, Mady V, Lefevre PC (1995) Development of two PCR assays for the identification of mycoplasmas causing contagious agalactia. FEMS Microbiol Lett 129:243-9

Dietz JP, Sertich PL, Boston RC, et al. Comparison of ticarcillin and piperacillin in Kenney's semen extender. Theriogenology. 2007;68(6):848–852.

Donn A, Jones GE, Ruiu A, Ladu M, Machell J, Stancanelli A (1997) Serological diagnosis of chlamydial abortion in sheep and goats: comparison of the complement fixation test and an enzyme-linked immunosorbent assay employing solubilised proteins as antigen.Vet Microbiol 59:27-36

Dunbar BS, Prasad SV, Timmons TM (1991) Comparative structure and function of mammalian zonae pellucidae in A comparative overview of mammalian fertilization ed. BS Dunbar and MG O'Rand NY Plenum press pp. 97-116

Eaglesome MD, Hare WCD and Singh EL (1980) Canadian Vet J 21: 106

Ellis WA (1994) Leptospirosis as a cause of reproductive failure Vet Clin North Am Food Anim Pract 10:463-78

Entrican G, Wilkie R, McWaters P, Scheerlinck J, Wood PR, Brown (1999) Cytokine release by ovine macrophages following infection with Chlamydia psittaci. J Clin Exp Immunol117:309-15

Everett KD, Andersen AA (1999) Identification of nine species of the Chlamydiaceae using PCR- RFLP.Int J Syst Bacteriol 49:803-13

Everett KD, Bush RM, Andersen AA (1999) Emended description of the order Chlamydiales, proposal of Parachlamydiaceae fam. nov. and Simkaniaceae fam. nov., each containing one monotypic genus, revised taxonomy of the family

Chlamydiaceae, including a new genus and five new species, and standards for the identification of organisms. Int J Syst Bacteriol 49:415-40

Farin, P. W., P. J. Chenoweth, D. F. Tomky, L. Ball, and J. E. Pexton. 1989. Breeding soundness, libido and performance of beef bulls mated to estrus synchronized females. Theriogenology 32: 717-725.

Farina R, Cerri D, Renzoni G, Andreani E, Mani P, Ebani V, Pedrini A, Nuvoloni R (1996) Leptospira interrogans in the genital tract of sheep. Research on ewes and rams experimentally infected with serovar hardjo (hardjobovis). New Microbiol 19:235-42

Fayrer-Hosken R, Christine Abreu-Barbosa, Gary Heusner, et al. Cryopreservation of stallion spermatozoa with INRA96 and glycerol. Journal of Equine Veterinary Science. 2008;28(11):672-676.

Feizabadi MM, Robertson ID, Hope A, Cousins DV, Hampson DJ (1997) Differentiation of Australian isolates of Mycobacterium paratuberculosis using pulsed-field gel electrophoresis Aust Vet J 75;887- 889

Feradis AH, Pawitri D, Suatha IK, et al. Cryopreservation of epididymal spermatozoa collected by needle biopsy from cynomolgus monkeys (Macaca fascicularis). J Med Primatol. 2001;30(2):100-106.

Foote RH. The history of artificial insemination: Selected notes and notables. Journal of Animal Science. 2002;80(E- Suppl 2):1-10.

Gao G.F, Hussain MH, Reid HW, Gould E.A (1994) Identification of naturally occurring monoclonal antibody escape variants of louping ill virus. J gen virol 75: 609-614.

Gao GF, Jiang WR, Hussain MH, Venugopal K, Gritsun TS, Reid HW, Gould EA (1993) Sequencing and antigenic studies of a Norwegian virus isolated from encephalomyelitic sheep confirm the existence of louping ill virus outside Great Britain and Ireland. Journal of General Virology 74: 109-114

Gao GF, Zanotto PM, de A, Holmes EC, Reid HW, Gould EA (1997) Molecular variation, evolution and geographical distribution of louping ill virus. Acta-Virologica. 41: 259-268

Garin-Bastuji B, Blasco JM, Grayon M, Verger JM (1998) Brucella melitensis infection in sheep: present and future Vet Res 29: 255-74

Gaumont R (1966) [Study of the presence of ant-leptospira agglutinins in domestic animals in France]. Bull Off Int Epizoot 66:833-48

Geering WA, Forman AJ and Nunn MJ (1995) Exotic diseases of animals-a field guide for Australian veterinarians Australian Government Publishing Service, Canberra

Georgsson G (1990) Maedi-visna pathology and pathogenesis in Maedi-visna and related diseases ed. G Petursson and R Hoff-Jorgensen Kluwer Academic Publishers pp.19-54

Gerritsen MA, Smits MA, Olyhoek T (1995) Random amplified polymorphic DNA fingerprinting for rapid identification of leptospiras of serogroup Sejroe. J Med Microbiol 42:336-9

Gibbs EPJ,Greiner EC (1994) The epidemiology of bluetongue Comp Immunol Microbiol Infect Dis 17:207-220

Gil, MC, Hermoso de Mendoza M, Rey J, Alonso JM, Poveda JB, Hermoso de Mendoza J (1999) Aretiology of caprine agalactia syndrome in Extramadura, Spain Vet Rec 144: 24-25

Gilbert, RO, Coubrough RI, Weiss KE (1987) The transmission of bluetongue virus by embryo transfer in sheep. Theriogenology 27: 527-540.

Gilmore and Angus (1991) Johne's disease in Sheep Diseases WB Martin and ID Aitken Blackwell Girjes AA, Hugall A, Graham DM, McCaul TF, Lavin MF (1993) Comparison of type I and type II

Gilmore JA, Liu J, Peter AT, et al. Determination of plasma membrane characteristics of boar spermatozoa and their relevance to cryopreservation. Biol Reprod. 1998;58(1):28-36.

Givens, M. D., J. A. Gard, and D. A. Stringfellow. 2007. Relative risks and approaches to biosecurity in the use of embryo technologies in livestock. Theriogenology 68: 298-307.

Glazebrook JS, Campbell RS, Hutchinson GW, Stallman ND (1978) Rodent zoonoses in North Queensland: the occurrence and distribution of zoonotic infections in North Queensland rodents. Aust J Exp Biol Med Sci Apr;56(2):147-56

Gordon LM (1980) Isolation of Leptospira interrogans serovar Hardjo from sheep Aust Vet J. 56:348- 9

Graham EF, Crabo BG, Pace MM. Current status of semen preservation in the ram, boar and stallion. Journal of Animal Science. 1978;47(Supplement II):80-119.

Greenwood PL, North RN, Kirkland PD (1995) Prevalence, spread and control of caprine arthritis- encephalitis virus in dairy goat herds in New South Wales AVJ 72:341-345.

Griffiths PC, Plater JM, Martin TC, Hughes SL, Hughes KJ, Hewinson RG, Dawson M (1995) Epizootic bovine abortion in a dairy herd: characterization of a Chlamydia psittaci isolate and antibody response. Br Vet J 151:683-93.

Grillo MJ, Barberan M and Blasco JM (1999) Experimental Brucella ovis infection in pregnant ewes. Vet Rec 144: 555-558.

Grillo MJ, Marin CM, Barberan M and Blasco JM (1997) Transmission of Brucella melitensis from sheep to lambs. Vet Rec 140: 602-605

Guerin B, Nibart M, Marquant-Le Guienne B, Humblot P (1997) Sanitary risks related to embryo transfer in domestic species. Theriogenology 47: 33-42.

Gunnersson E and Fodstad FH (1979) Cultural and biochemical characteristics of Mycobacterium paratuberculosis isolated from goats in Norway Acta Veterinaria Scand 20: 122-134.

Gut-Zangger P, Vretou E, Psarrou E, Pospischil A, Thoma R (1999) [No title available]. Schweiz Arch Tierheilkd;141:361-6.

Gwozdz JM, Reichel MP, Murray A, Manktelow W, West DM, Thompson KG (1997) Detection of Mycobacterium avium subsp. paratuberculosis in ovine tissues and blood by the polymerase chain reaction. Vet Microbiol 57: 233-244.

Harbi MSMA, El-Tahir MS, Salim MO, Nayil AA, Mageed IA (1983) Experimental contagious caprine pleuropneumonia Goat diseases, Mycoplasma mycoides. Trop Anim Health Prod. Edinburgh : Longman. 15: 51-52.

Hare WCD, Luedke AJ, Thomas FC, Bowen RA, Singh EL, Eaglesome MD, Randall GCB, Bielanski A (1988) Non-transmission of bluetongue virus by embryos from bluetongue virus-infected sheep. Amer. J Vet Res. 49: 468-472

Hathaway SC, Little TW, Stevens AE, Ellis WA, Morgan J (1983) Serovar identification of leptospires of the Australis serogroup isolated from free-living and domestic species in the United Kingdom. Res Vet Sci 35:64-8

He S, Woods LC. Effects of glycine and alanine on short-term storage and cryopreservation of striped bass (Morone saxatilis) spermatozoa. Cryobiology. 2003;46(1):17-25.

Heape W. The artificial insemination of mammals and subsequent possible fertilization or impregnation of their ova. Proceedings of the Royal Society of London. 1987;B(61):52-63.

Hecht SJ, Sharp JM, Demartini JC (1996) Retroviral aetiopathogenesis of ovine pulmonary carcinoma: a critical appraisal. Br Vet J 152:395-409.

Heinemann MB, Garcia JF, Nunes CM, Morais ZM, Gregori F, Cortez A, Vasconcellos SA, Visintin JA, Richtzenhain LJ (1999) Detection of leptospires in bovine semen by polymerase chain reaction. Aust Vet J 77:32-4.

Herr S (1994) Brucella melitensis infection in Infectious diseases of livestock with special reference to South Africa JAW Coetzer, GR Thomson, RC Tustin (eds.) Oxford pp 1073-1075.

Hod I, Perk K, Nobel TA, Klopfer U (1972) Lung carcinoma of sheep (Jaagsiekte), III Lymph node, blood, and immunoglobulin J Natl Cancer Instit 48: 487-507.

Hoffmann B, Landeck A. Testicular endocrine function, seasonality and semen quality of the stallion. Anim Reprod Sci. 1999;57(1-2):89-98.

Hoffmann N, Oldenhof H, Morandini C, et al. Optimal concentrations of cryoprotective agents for semen from stallions that are classified 'good' or 'poor' for freezing. Animal Reproduction Science. 2011;125(1-4):112-118.

Holland MJ, Palmarini M, Garcia-Goti M, Gonzalez L, McKendrick I, de las Heras M, Sharp JM (1999) Jaagsiekte retrovirus is widely distributed both in T and B lymphocytes and in mononuclear phagocytes of sheep with naturally and experimentally acquired pulmonary adenomatosis. J Virol 73:4004-8.

Holt WV. Basic aspects of frozen storage of semen. Anim Reprod Sci. 2000;62(1-3):3-22.

Holtz, W., B. Sohnrey, M. Gerland, and M. A. Driancourt. 2008. Ovsynch synchronization and fixed-time insemination in goats. Theriogenology 69: 785-792.

Houwers DJ (1990) Economic importance, epidemiology and control in Maedi-Visna and related diseases ed. G Petursson and R Hoff-Jorgensen Kluwer Academic Publishers pp. 83-117.

Houwers DJ and Terpestra C (1984) Sheep pulmonary adenomatosis Vet Rec 114: 23.

Houwers DJ, Konig CD, Bakker J, de Boer MJ, Pekelder JJ, Sol J, Vellema P, de Vries G (1987)

Houwers DJ, van der Molen EJ (1987) A five-year serological study of natural transmission of maedi-visna virus in a flock of sheep, completed with post mortem examination. J Vet Med. B 34: 421-431

Houwers DJ, Visscher AH and Defize PR (1989) Importance of ewe/lamb relationship and breed in the epidemiology of maedi-visna virus infections. Res Vet Science 46:5-8.

Hubalek Z; Pow I; Reid HW; Hussain MH (1995) Antigenic similarity of Central European encephalitis and louping-ill viruses. Acta-Virologica. 39: 251-256.

Huchzermeyer HFAK, Bruckner GK, Bastianello SS (1994) Paratuberculosis in Infectious diseases of livestock with special reference to South Africa JAW Coetzer, GR Thomson, RC Tustin (eds.) Oxford pp 1445-1457

Hunter AR and Munro R (1983) The diagnosis, occurrence and distribution of sheep pulmonary adenomatosis in Scotland. Brit Vet J 139: 153-164

Hutber AM, Kitching RP, Conway DA (1999) Predicting the level of herd infection for outbreaks of foot- and-mouth disease in vaccinated herds. Epidemiol Infect 122: 539-44

Ireland DC and Binepal YS (1998) Improved detection of capripoxvirus in biopsy samples by PCR. J Virol Methods 74: 1-7

Jeggo M, Wright P, Anderson J, Eaton B, Afshar A, Pearson J, Kirkland P, Ozawa Y (1992) Review of the IAEA meeting in Vienna on standardisation of the competitive ELISA test and reagents for the diagnosis of bluetongue in Bluetongue, African horse sickness and related orbiviruses Proceedings of the second international symposium eds. Walton TE and Osburn BI CRC Press 547- 560

Jimenez de bagues MP (1994) Vaccination with Brucella abortus rough mutant RB51 protects BALB/c mice against virulent strains of Brucella abortus, Brucella melitensis, and Brucella ovis. Infect Immun. 62:4990-6.

Joag SV, Stephens EB, Narayan O (1996) Lentiviruses in Fields virology, third edition ed. BN Fields, DM Kapie, PM Howley et al. Lippincott- Raven Publishers, Philadelphia, pp. 1977-1999

Jones GE (1997) Guest editorial; Chlamydial disease-More than just abortion Vet J 153 249-251

Kaiser R, Kern A, Kampa D, Neumann-Haefelin D (1997) Prevalence of antibodies to Borrelia burgdorferi and tick-borne encephalitis virus in an endemic region in southern Germany. Zentralbl Bakteriol 286:534-41

Kajikawa O, Dahlberg JE, Rosadio RH, De Martini JC (1990) Detection and quantitation of a type D retrovirus gag protein in ovine pulmonary carcinoma (sheep pulmonary adenomatosis) by means of a competition radioimmunoassay. Vet Microbiol 25:17-28

Kaltenboeck B, Heard D, DeGraves FJ, Schmeer N J (1997) Use of synthetic antigens improves detection by enzyme-linked immunosorbent assay of antibodies against abortigenic Chlamydia psittaci in ruminants. Clin Microbiol 35:2293-8

Kapoor SG, Singh PP, Pathak RC (1983) Prevalence of Mycoplasma/Acholeplsma in the genital tract of goats Indian J Comp Microbiol, Immunol and Infectious dis. 4:102-106

Kareskoski M, Katila T. Components of stallion seminal plasma and the effects of seminal plasma on sperm longevity. Animal Reproduction Science. 2008;107(3-4):249-256.

Kennedy DJ (1999) Progress in National Control and Assurance programs for Bovine Johne's Disease in Australia. Sixth International Colloquium on Paratuberculosis Melbourne, Abstract pp. 24.

Kinde H, DaMassa AIj, Wakenell PS, Petty R (1994) Mycoplasma infection in a commercial goat dairy caused by Mycoplasma agalactia and Mycoplasma mycoides subsp. mycoides (caprine biotype) J Vet Diagn Invest 6: 423-427

Kirkbride CA, Johnson MW (1989) Serologic examination of aborted ovine and bovine fetal fluids for the diagnosis of border disease, bluetongue, bovine viral diarrhea, and leptospiral infections. J Vet Diagn Invest 1:132-8

Kitching RP, Taylor WP (1985) Transmission of capripoxvirus. Research in Veterinary-Science. 39: 196-199

Koskinen E, Junnila M, Katila T, et al. A preliminary study on the use of betaine as a cryoprotective agent in deep freezing of stallion semen. Journal of Veterinary Medicine Series A. 1989;36(1-10):110-114.

Koumbati M, Mangana O, Nomikou K, Mellor PS, Papadopoulos O (1999) Duration of bluetongue viraemia and serological responses in experimentally infected European breeds of sheep and goats Vet Microbiol 64:277-85

Kraemer, D. C. 1989. Embryo collection and transfer in small ruminants. Theriogenology 31: 141-148.

Kwang J, Keen J, Roast S and Toiler F (1995) Development and application of an antibody ELISA for the marker protein of ovine pulmonary carcinoma. Vet Immunol and Immunoparasitol 47: 323-331

Lamb, G. C., C. R. Dahlen, J. E. Larson, G. Marquezini, and J. S. Stevenson. 2010. Control of the estrous cycle to improve fertility for fixed-time artificial insemination in beef cattle: a review. J Anim Sci 88: E181-192.

Larson, J. E., K. N. Thielen, B. J. Funnell, J. S. Stevenson, D. J. Kesler, and G. C. Lamb. 2009. Influence of a controlled internal drug release after fixed-time artificial insemination on pregnancy rates and returns to estrus of nonpregnant cows. J Anim Sci 87: 914-921.

Leach RH, Erna H, MacOwan KJ (1993) Proposal for designation of F38-type caprine mycoplasmas as Mycoplasma capricolum subsp. capripneumoniae subsp. nov. and consequent obligatory relegation of strains currently classified as M. capricolum (Tully, Barile, Edward, Theodore, and Erno 1974) to an additional new subspecies, Mycoplasma capricolum subsp. capricolum subsp. nov Int J Syst Bacteriol 43: 603-605

Leon-Vizcaino L, Hermoso de Mendoza M, Garrido F (1987) Incidence of abortions caused by leptospirosis in sheep and goats in Spain. Comp Immunol Microbiol Infect Dis;10:149-53

Levisohn S., Davidson I., Caro Vergara M.-R. & Rapaport E. (1991). Use of an ELISA for differential diagnosis of Mycoplasma agalactiae and M. mycoides subsp. mycoides LC in naturally infected goat herds. Res. Vet. Sci. 51, 66-71.

Liao YK, Chain CY, Lu YS, Li NJ, Tsai HJ, Liou PP (1997) Epizootic of Chlamydia psittaci infection in goats in Taiwan. J Basic Microbiol; 37:327-33

Light MR, Schipper IA, Molitor TW, Tilton JE and Slanger WD (1979) Progressive pneumonia in sheep: incidence of natural infection and establishment of clean flocks J Anim Sc 49: 1157-1160

Little TW, Stevens AE, Hathaway SC (1987) Serological studies of British leptospiral isolates of the Sejroe serogroup. III. The distribution of leptospires of the Sejroe serogroup in the British Isles Epidemiol Infect 99:117-26

Loomis PR, Graham JK. Commercial semen freezing: Individual male variation in cryosurvival and the response of stallion sperm to customized freezing protocols. Anim Reprod Sci. 2008;105(1-2):119-128.

Lujan L, Badiola JJ, Garcia-Marin JF, Moreno B, Vargas MA, Fernandez de Luco D, Perez V (1993) Seroprevalence of maedi-visna infection in sheep in the north-east of Spain. Preventive Veterinary Medicine. 15: 181-190

MacCaughan CJ, Gordon LM and Rahaley RS (1980) Evidence for infection of sheep in Victoria with leptospires of the hebdomadis group Aust Vet J 56:201-202.

Macías García B, Ortega Ferrusola C, Aparicio IM, et al. Toxicity of glycerol for the stallion spermatozoa: effects on membrane integrity and cytoskeleton, lipid peroxidation and mitochondrial membrane potential. Theriogenology. 2012;77(7):1280-1289.

MacOwan KJ and Minette JE (1977) Contact transmission of experimental contagious pleuropneumonia (CCPP). Trop Anim Health Prod 9:185-188

MacOwan KJ and Minette JE (1978) The effect of high passage mycoplasma strain F38 on the course of contagious caprine pleuropneumonia (CCPP). Trop Anim Health Prod 10: 31-35

Maedi-visna control in sheep. III: Results and evaluation of a voluntary control program in The Netherlands over a period of four years. Vet Q Nov;9 Suppl 1:29S-36S

Mangana-Vougiouka O, Markoulatos P, Koptopoulos G, Nomikou K, Bakandritsos N, Papadopoulos O J (1999) Sheep poxvirus identification by PCR in cell cultures Virol Methods 77: 75-9

Mann JA, Seller RF (1990) Foot and mouth disease in Virus infections of ruminant ed. Z Dinter and B Morein, Elsevier pp.503-512

Marco J, Gonzalez L, Cuervo LA, Beltran de Heredia F, Barberan M, Marin C, Blasco JM (1994) Brucella ovis infection in two flocks of sheep. Vet Rec 10:254-6

Mare CJ (1994) Contagious caprine pleuropneumonia in Infectious diseases of livestock with special reference to South Africa JAW Coetzer, GR Thomson, RC Tustin (eds.) Oxford pp 1495-1497

Marin MS, McKenzie J, Gao GF, Reid HW, Antoiadis A, Gould EA (1995) The virus causing encephalomyelitis in sheep in Spain: a new member of the tick-borne encephalitis group. Res Vet Science 58: 11-13

Marin MS, McKenzie J, Gao GF, Reid HW, Antoniadis A, Gould EA (1995) The virus causing encephalomyelitis in sheep in Spain: a new member of the tick-borne encephalitis group. Res Vet Sci 58:11-13

Mayr A and Czerny CP (1990) Cowpox virus in Virus infections of ruminants (ed.) Z Dinter and B Morein Elsevier Science pp. 9-16

McGann LE. Differing actions of penetrating and nonpenetrating cryoprotective agents. Cryobiology. 1978;15(4):382–390.

McKenzie J (1991) Survey for caprine arthritis encephalitis antibodies in sheep Surveillance 18:19-20

Mebus CA, Singh EL (1988) Failure to transmit foot-and-mouth disease via bovine embryo transfer. Proc. U.S. Animal Health Assoc 92: 183-185.

Melican, D., and W. Gavin. 2008. Repeat superovulation, non-surgical embryo recovery, and surgical embryo transfer in transgenic dairy goats. Theriogenology 69: 197-203.

Mellor PS, Boorman J (1995) The transmission and geographical spread of African horse sickness and bluetongue viruses. Ann Trop Med Parasitol 89:1-15

Menchaca, A., M. Vilarino, M. Crispo, T. de Castro, and E. Rubianes. 2010. New approaches to

Merza M and Mushi EZ (1990) Sheep pox virus in Virus infections of ruminants (ed.) Z Dinter and B Morein Elsevier Science pp. 43-48

Monath TP and Heinz FX (1996) Flaviviruses in Fields Virology Third Edition, ed. BN Fields, DM Knipe, PM Howley et al. Lippincott-Raven Publishers, Philadelphia

Moore AI, Squires EL, Graham JK. Adding cholesterol to the stallion sperm plasma membrane improves cryosurvival. Cryobiology. 2005;51(3):241–249.

Moulton JE (1990) Tumours of the respiratory system in Tumours in domestic animals 3rd edition ed. JE Moulton. University of California Press pp.308-346

Munz E and Dumbell K (1994) Sheeppox and goatpox in Infectious diseases of livestock with special reference to South Africa JAW Coetzer, GR Thomson, RC Tustin (eds.) Oxford pp.613-615.

Muthomi EK, Rurangirwa FR (1983). Passive haemagglutination and complement fixation as diagnostic tests for contagious caprine pleuropneumonia caused by the F38 strain mycoplasma. Res. Vet. Sci. 35: 1- 4.

Mycoplasma agalactia. Cornell Vet 64: 435-442

Mycoplasma bovigenitalium with preimplantation bovine embryos. Theriogenology 32: 633-641

Narayan O, Cork LC (1990) Caprine arthritis-encephalitis virus in Virus infections of ruminants ed. Z Dinter and B Morein, Elsevier, Amsterdam, pp. 441-452

Narayan O, Griffin DE, Chase J (1977) Antigenic shift of visna virus in a persistently infected sheep. Science 197: 376-378

Nord K, Holstad G, Eik LO, Gronstol H (1998) Control of caprine arthritis-encephalitis virus and Corynebacterium pseudotuberculosis infection in a Norwegian goat herd Acta Vet Scand 39:109-17

O'Flaherty CM, Beorlegui NB, Beconi MT. Reactive oxygen species requirements for bovine sperm capacitation and acrosome reaction. Theriogenology. 1999;52(2):289-301.

Oldenhof H, Gojowsky M, Wang S, et al. Osmotic Stress and Membrane Phase Changes During Freezing of Stallion Sperm: Mode of Action of Cryoprotective Agents. Biol Reprod. 2013;88(3):68.

Oliver RE, Gorham JR, Parish SF, Hadlow WT, Narayan O (1981) Ovine progressive pneumonia; pathologic and virologic studies on the naturally occurring disease Am J Vet Res 42: 1554- 1559

Omotese, B. O., P. I. Rekwot, H. J. Makun, J. A. Obidi, J. S. Rwuaan, and N. P. Chiezey. 2010. Evaluation of EAZI-Breed CIDR and FGA-30 intravaginal sponge as estrus synchronizing agents in pre-partum red sokoto does. Veterinary Research 3: 64-69.

Ortin A, Minguijon E, Dewar P, Garcia M, Ferrer LM, Palmarini M, Gonzalez L, Sharp JM, De las Heras M (1998) Lack of a specific immune response against a recombinant capsid protein of Jaagsiekte sheep retrovirus in sheep and goats naturally affected by enzootic nasal tumour or sheep pulmonary adenomatosis. Vet Immunol Immunopathol 61:229-37

Osburn BI (1994) The impact of bluetongue virus on reproduction. Comp Immunol Microbiol Infect Dis 17:189-96

Pagl R, Aurich JE, Müller-Schlösser F, et al. Comparison of an extender containing defined milk protein fractions with a skim milk-based extender for storage of equine semen at 5°C. Theriogenology. 2006;66(5):1115-1122.

Palit A, Haylock LM, Cox JC (1986) Storage of pathogenic leptospires in liquid nitrogen J Appl Bacteriol 61:407-11

Palmarini M, Holland MJ, Cousens C, Dalziel RG, Sharp JM (1996) Jaagsiekte retrovirus establishes a disseminated infection of the lymphoid tissues of sheep affected by pulmonary adenomatosis J gen virol 77: 2991- 2998

Palmarini M, Sharp JM, de las Heras M, Fan H (1999) Jaagsiekte sheep retrovirus is necessary and sufficient to induce a contagious lung cancer in sheep.J Virol 73:6964-72

Papa FO, Felício GB, Melo-Oña CM, et al. Replacing egg yolk with soybean lecithin in the cryopreservation of stallion semen. Animal Reproduction Science. 2011;129(1-2):73-77.

Papadopoulos O, Paschaleri-Papadopoulos E, Deligaris N, Doukas G (1971) [Isolation of tick-borne encephalitis virus from a flock of goats with abortions and fatal disease (a preliminary report)]. Kteniatrika-Nea. 3: 112-114.

Parker BNJ, Wrathall AE, Saunders, RW, Dawson M, Done SH, Francis PG, Dexter I, Bradley R (1998) Prevention of transmission of sheep pulmonary adenomatosis by embryo transfer. Vet Rec 142:687-689.

Pasick J (1998) Use of a recombinant maedi-visna virus protein ELISA for the serologic diagnosis of lentivirus infections in small ruminants. Can J Vet Res 62: 307-310

Pay TWF (1988) Foot-and mouth disease in sheep and goats: A review Foot and Mouth Disease Bulletin 26: 2-13

Pegg DE. The history and principles of cryopreservation. Semin Reprod Med. 2002;20(1):5-13.

Peña FJ, García BM, Samper JC, et al. Dissecting the molecular damage to stallion spermatozoa: the way to improve current cryopreservation protocols? Theriogenology. 2011;76(7):1177-1186.

Pereira, R. J., B. Sohnrey, and W. Holtz. 1998. Nonsurgical embryo collection in goats treated with prostaglandin F2alpha and oxytocin. J Anim Sci 76: 360-363.

Perez V, Tellechea J, Badiola JJ, Gutierrez M, Garcia Marin JF (1997) Relation between serologic response and pathologic findings in sheep with naturally acquired paratuberculosis. Am J Vet Res 58: 799- 803

Perreau P Le Goff C. & Giauffret A. (1976). Le diagnostic sérologique de l'agalactie contagieuse des petits ruminants : un test de fixation du complément. Bull. Acad. Vét. Fr., 49, 185-192.

Petursson G (1990) Maedi-visna. Etiology and immune response in Maedi-visna and related diseases ed. G Petursson and R Hoff-Jorgensen Kluwer Academic Publishers pp.55-71

Pexton, J. E., P. W. Farin, R. A. Gerlach, J. L. Sullins, M. C. Shoop, and P. J. Chenoweth. 1989. Efficiency of single-sire mating programs with beef bulls mated to estrus synchronized females. Theriogenology 32: 705-716.

Philpott M (1993) The dangers of disease transmission by artificial insemination and embryo transfer. Brit vet J 149: 339-369

Pillet E, Duchamp G, Batellier F, et al. Egg yolk plasma can replace egg yolk in stallion freezing extenders. Theriogenology. 2011;75(1):105-114.

Pillet E, Labbe C, Batellier F, et al. Liposomes as an alternative to egg yolk in stallion freezing extender. Theriogenology. 2012;77(2):268-279.

Plant JW, Beh KJ, Acland HM (1972) Laboratory findings from ovine abortion and perinatal mortality Aust Vet J 48: 558-561

Pojprasath T, Lohachit C, Techakumphu M, et al. Improved cryo-preservability of stallion sperm using a sorbitol-based freezing extender. Theriogenology. 2011;75(9):1742-1749.

Pukazhenthi BS, Johnson A, Guthrie HD, et al. Improved sperm cryosurvival in diluents containing amides versus glycerol in the Przewalski's horse (Equus ferus przewalskii). Cryobiology. 2014;68(2):205-214.

Pukazhenthi BS, Togna GD, Padilla L, et al. Ejaculate Traits and Sperm Cryopreservation in the Endangered Baird's Tapir (Tapirus bairdii). Journal of Andrology. 2011;32(3):260-270.

Ramón M, Pérez-Guzmán MD, Jiménez-Rabadán P, et al. Sperm cell population dynamics in ram remen during the cryopreservation process. PLoS ONE. 2013;8(3):e59189.

Rao TV, Malik P, Nandi S, Negi BS (1997) Evaluation of immunocapture ELISA for diagnosis of goat pox. Acta Virol 1: 345-8

Rathbone, M. J., K. L. Macmillan, W. Jochle, M. P. Boland, and E. K. Inskeep. 1998. Controlled-release products for the control of the estrus cycle in cattle, sheep, goats, deer, pigs, and horses. Critical Reviews in Therapeutic Drug Carrier Systems 15: 285-379.

Reddington JJ, Reddington GM, MacLachlan NJ (1991) A competitive ELISA for detection of antibodies to the group antigen of bluetongue virus. J Vet Diagn Inves, 3, 144-147

Reid HW and Doherty PC (1971) Louping ill encephalomyelitis in the sheep 1. The relationship of viraemia and the antibody response to susceptibility. J Comp Pathol 81: 521-530

Reid HW; Buxton D; Pow I; Finlayson J (1984) Transmission of louping-ill virus in goat milk. Vet Rec. 114: 163-165

Renard P, Grizard G, Griveau JF, et al. Improvement of motility and fertilization potential of post thaw human sperm using glutamine. Cryobiology. 1996;33(3):311-319.

Ricker JV, Linfor JJ, Delfino WJ, et al. Equine sperm membrane phase behavior: the effects of lipid-based cryoprotectants. Biol Reprod. 2006;74(2):359-365.

Riddell KP, Stringfellow DA and Panaangala VS (1989b) Interaction of Mycoplasma bovis and

Riddell KP, Stringfellow DA, Wolfe DF and Galik PK (1989a) In vitro exposure of ovine ova to Brucella abortus. Theriogenology 31: 895-901

Riddell KP, Stringfellow DA, Wolfe DF and Galik PK (1990) Seroconversion of recipient ewes after transfer of embryos exposed to Brucella ovis in vitro. Theriogenology 34: 965-973.

Roberts DH, Lucas MH, Bell RA (1993) Animal and animal product importation and the assessment of risk from bluetongue and other ruminant orbiviruses. Br Vet J 149: 87-99.

Roca, J., J. M. Vazquez, M. A. Gil, C. Cuello, I. Parrilla, and E. A. Martinez. 2006. Challenges in pig artificial insemination. Reproduction in Domestic Animals 41 Suppl 2: 43-53.

Rocha T (1998) A review of leptospirosis in farm animals in Portugal. Rev Sci Tech Dec;17:699-712.

Rohde RF; Shulaw WP; Hueston WD; Bech Nielsen S; Haibel GK; Hoffsis GF (1990) Isolation of Mycobacterium paratuberculosis from washed bovine ova after in vitro exposure. Am J Vet Res 51:708-710.

Ros Bascunana C, Mattson JG, Bolske G, Johansson KE (1994) Characterisation of the 16S rRNA genes from Mycoplasma sp. strain F38 and development of an identification system based on PCR. J Bacteriol 176: 2577-2586

Rosati S, Kwang J, Tolari F, Keen J (1994) A comparison of whole virus and recombinant transmembrane ELISA and immunodiffusion for detection of ovine lentivirus antibodies in Italian sheep flocks. Veterinary- Research-Communications. 18: 73-80.

Rosati S, Pittau M, Alberti A, Pozzi S, York DF, Sharp JM, Palmarini M (2000) An accessory open reading frame (orf-x) of jaagsiekte sheep retrovirus is conserved between different virus isolates. Virus Res 66:109-16

Roy, F., B. Combes, D. Vaiman, E. P. Cribiu, T. Pobel, F. Deletang, Y. Combarnous, F. Guillou, and M. C. Maurel. 1999a. Humoral immune response to equine chorionic gonadotropin in ewes: association with major histocompatibility complex and interference with subsequent fertility. Biol Reprod 61: 209-218.

Roy, F., M. C. Maurel, B. Combes, D. Vaiman, E. P. Cribiu, I. Lantier, T. Pobel, F. Deletang, Y. Combarnous, and F. Guillou. 1999b. The negative effect of repeated equine chorionic gonadotropin treatment on subsequent fertility in Alpine goats is due to a humoral immune response involving the major histocompatibility complex. Biol Reprod 60: 805-813.

Royere D, Barthelemy C, Hamamah S, et al. Cryopreservation of spermatozoa: a 1996 review. Human Reproduction Update. 1996;2(6):553-559.

Rubianes, E., and A. Menchaca. 2003. The pattern and manipulation of ovarian follicular growth in goats. Animal Reproduction Science 78: 271-287.

Salamon S, Maxwell WM. Storage of ram semen. Anim Reprod Sci. 2000;62(1-3):77-111.

Salinas J, Souriau A, Cuello F, Rodolakis A (1995) Antigenic diversity of ruminant Chlamydia psittaci strains demonstrated by the indirect microimmunofluorescence test with monoclonal antibodies Vet Microbiol 43: 219-226

Salinas-Flores L, Adams SL, Lim MH. Determination of the membrane permeability characteristics of pacific oyster, Crassostrea gigas, oocytes and development of optimized methods to add and remove ethylene glycol. Cryobiology. 2008;56(1):43–52.

Saman E, Van Eynde G, Lujan L, Extramiana B, Harkiss G, Tolari F, Gonzalez L, Amorena B, Watt N, Badiola (1999) A new sensitive serological assay for detection of lentivirus infections in small ruminants. J Clin Diagn Lab Immunol 6:734-40

Sanches EG, Oliveira IR, Serralheiro PC, et al. Cryopreservation of mutton snapper (Lutjanus analis) sperm. Anais da Academia Brasileira de Ciências. 2013;85(3):1083–1092.

Sánchez-Partida LG, Maxwell WM, Paleg LG, et al. Proline and glycine betaine in cryoprotective diluents for ram spermatozoa. Reprod Fertil Dev. 1992;4(1):113–118.

Scharp DW, al Khalaf SA, al Muhanna MW, Cheema RA, Godana W (1999) Use of mass vaccination with a reduced dose of REV 1 vaccine for Brucella melitensis control in a population of small ruminants. Trop Anim Health Prod 31:135-41

Schmitz JA, Coles BM, Shires GM (1981) Fatal hemolytic disease in sheep attributed to Leptospira interrogans serotype hardjo infection. Cornell Vet 71:175-82

Seaman JT (1985) Chlamydia isolated from abortion in sheep AustVet J 62:436

Sharma SK (1978) Studies on foot-and-mouth disease in sheep with special reference to distribution of the virus and carrier state. Vet Res Bull 1: 156-157.

Sharma SK, Murty DK (1981) Foot-and-mouth disease in sheep: pattern of virus excretion and distribution in the experimentally infected animals. Indian Journal of Animal Sciences. 51: 61-66.

Sharp JM, Angus KW, Jassim FA, Scott FMM (1986) Experimental transmission of sheep pulmonary adenomatosis to a goat. Vet Rec 119: 245

Shin, S. T., S. K. Jang, H. S. Yang, O. K. Lee, Y. H. Shim, W. I. Choi, D. S. Lee, G. S. Lee, J. K. Cho, and Y. W. Lee. 2008. Laparoscopy vs. laparotomy for embryo transfer to produce transgenic goats (Capra hircus). Journal of Veterinary Science 9: 103-107.

Si W, Zheng P, Li Y, et al. Effect of glycerol and dimethyl sulfoxide on cryopreservation of rhesus monkey (Macaca mulatta) sperm. Am J Primatol. 2004;62(4):301–306.

Sihvonen L (1980) Studies on transmission of maedi virus to lambs. Acta Vet Scandinavica 21: 689-698.

Simard CL, Briscoe MR (1990) An enzyme-linked immunosorbent assay for detection of antibodies to maedi-visna virus in sheep. A simple technique for production of antigen using sodium dodecyl sulfate treatment. Can. J. Vet. Res. 54, 446-450.

Singh EL, Dulac GC, Henderson JM (1997) Embryo transfer as a means of controlling the transmission of viral infections. XV. Failure to transmit bluetongue virus through the transfer of embryos from viraemic sheep donors. Theriogenology. 47: 1205-1214.

Singh N, Rajya BS, Mohanty GC (1974) Granular vulvo-vaginitis (GVV) in goats associated with

Smith GP II. Through a test tube darkly: artificial insemination and the law. Michigan Law Review. 1968;67(1):127-150.

Smith VW, Dickson J, Coackley W, Carman H (1985) Response of merino sheep to inoculation with a caprine retrovirus. Vet Rec 117: 61-3

Snoeck PPN, Cottorello ACP, Henry M. Viability and fertility of stallion semen frozen with ethylene glycol and acetamide as a cryogenic agent. Animal Reproduction Science. 2012;9(1):33-39.

Snowder GD, Gates NL, Glimp HA, Gorham JR (1990) Prevalence and effect of subclinical ovine progressive pneumonia virus infection on ewe wool and lamb production. J Am Vet Med Assoc 197:475-9

Snowdon WA (1968) The susceptibility of some Australian fauna to infection with foot-and-mouth disease virus. Aust Jnl Exp Med Sci 46: 667

Sohnrey, B., and W. Holtz. 2005. Technical Note: Transcervical deep cornual insemination of goats. J Anim Sci 83: 1543-1548.

Squires EL, Keith SL, Graham JK. Evaluation of alternative cryoprotectants for preserving stallion spermatozoa. Theriogenology. 2004;62(6):1056-1165.

Srinivas RP, Rajasekhar M (1992) Foot and mouth disease in sheep and goats Livestock adviser 17: 3- 9

Standfast HA, Dyce AL, Muller MJ (1985) Vectors of bluetongue virus in Australia in Bluetongue and related orbiviruses Alan R.Liss inc. pp 177-186

Storz J, Carroll EJ, Stephenson EH, Ball L, Eugster AK (1976) Urogenital infection and seminal excretion after inoculation of bulls and rams with chlamydiae Am J Vet Res 37: 517-520

Stringfellow DA (1998) Recommendations for the sanitary handling of in-vivo-derived embryos in Manual of the International Embryo Transfer Society DA Stringfellow and SM Seidel (eds.) 3rd edition, Internationa Embryo Transfer Society, Illinois, USA, pp. 79-84

Stringfellow, D. A., and M. D. Givens. 2000. Epidemiologic concerns relative to in vivo and in vitro production of livestock embryos. Animal Reproduction Science 60-61: 629-642.

superovulation and embryo transfer in small ruminants. Reprod Fertil Dev 22: 113-118.

Swanepoel R (1994) Louping ill in Infectious diseases of livestock with special reference to Southern Africa ed. JAW Coetzer, GR Thomson, RC Tustin Oxford university press Vol 1 pp671-677

Tabachnick WJ, Mellor PS, Standfast HA (1991) Working team report on vectors: recommendations for research on Culicoides vector biology in Bluetongue, African horse sickness and related orboviruses, Proceedings of the second international symposium ed. TE Waltonand BI Osburn CRC Press pp 977-989

Taylor K, Bashiruddin JB, Gould AR (1992) Relationships between members of the Mycoplasma mycoides cluster as shown by DNA probes and sequence analysis. Int J.Systematic Bact 42: 593-

Thibier M, Guerin B (1999) Embryo transfer in small ruminants: the method of choice for health control in germplasm exchanges in Livestock Production Science, Special issue "Reproductive Biotechnologies and disease control" (In press).

Thurston LM, Siggins K, Mileham AJ, et al. Identification of amplified restriction fragment length polymorphism markers linked to genes controlling boar sperm viability following cryopreservation. Biol Reprod. 2002;66(3):545-554.

Tian Y, Qi W, Jiang J, et al. Sperm cryopreservation of sex-reversed seven-band grouper, Epinephelus septem fasciatus. Animal Reproduction Science. 2013;137(3-4):230-236.

Tischner M. Evaluation of deep-frozen semen in stallions. J Reprod Fertil Suppl 1979;27:53-59.

Tola S, Angioi A, Rocchigiani AM, Idini G, Manunta D, Galleri G, Leori G (1997) Detection of Mycoplasma agalactiae in sheep milk samples by polymerase chain reaction. Vet Microbiol Jan:54:17- 22

Tola S, Idini G, Manunta D, Galleri G, Angioi A, Rocchigiani AM, Leori G (1996) Rapid and specific detection of Mycoplasma agalactiae by polymerase chain reaction. Vet Microbiol 51:77-84

Travassos C, Benoit C, Valas S, da Silva A, Perrin G (1998) [Detection of caprine arthritis encephalitis virus in sperm of experimentally infected bucks].[Article in French] Vet Res 29:579-84

Trimeche A, Yvon JM, Vidament M, et al. Effects of glutamine, proline, histidine and betaine on post-thaw motility of stallion spermatozoa. Theriogenology. 1999;52(1):181-191.

USDA-ERS. 2013. Farm milk production. USDA Economic Research Service, http://www.ers.usda.gov/topics/animal-products/dairy/background.aspx#milk.

Van Tonder EM, Herr S, Bishop GC, Bosman PP (1996) Brucella ovis infection in Infectious diseases of livestock with special reference to Southern Africa JAW Coetzer, GR Thomson, RC Tustin (eds.) Oxford University Press, Southern Africa, Capetown, Volume 2, pp 1065-1072

Verwoerd DW (1996) Guest editorial - Ovine pulmonary adenomatosis (jaagsiekte) Brit Vet J 152: 369- 372

Verwoerd DW, Tustin RC (1994) Caprine arthritis-encephalitis in Infectious Diseases of Livestock with special reference to Southern Africa. Coetzer JAW, Thomson GR, Tustin (eds.) Oxford University Press, Southern Africa, Capetown. Volume 2, pp. 797-799

Vidament M, Dupere AM, Julienne P, et al. Equine frozen semen: Freezability and fertility field results. Theriogenology. 1997;48(6):907-917.

Vishwanath R, Shannon P. Storage of bovine semen in liquid and frozen state. Animal Reproduction Science. 2000;62(1-3):23-53.

Vretou E, Loutrari H, Mariani L, Costelidou K, Eliades P, Conidou G, Karamanou S, Mangana O, Siarkou V, Papadopoulos O (1996) Diversity among abortion strains of Chlamydia psittaci demonstrated by inclusion morphology, polypeptide profiles and monoclonal antibodies. Vet Microbiol 51:275-89

Wade-Evans AM, Mertens PPC, Bostock CJ (1990) Development of the polymerase chain reaction for the detection of bluetongue virus in tissue samples J Virol Methods, 30, 15-24

Wagter LH, Jansen A, Bleumink-Pluym NM, Lenstra JA, Houwers DJ (1998) PCR detection of lentiviral GAG segment DNA in the white blood cells of sheep and goats. Vet Res Commun 22:355-62

Watson PF. The causes of reduced fertility with cryopreserved semen. Anim Reprod Sci. 2000;60-61:481-492.

Wesonga HO, Lindberg R, Litamoi JK, Bolske G (1998) Late lesions of experimental contagious caprine pleuropneumonia caused by Mycoplasma capricolum ssp. capripneumoniae. Zentralbl Veterinarmed 45:105-14

Whitley, N. C., and D. J. Jackson. 2004. An update on estrus synchronization in goats: a minor species. J Anim Sci 82 E-Suppl: E270-276.

Whittington RJ, Marsh I, McAllister S, Turner MJ, Marshall DJ, Fraser CA (1999) Evaluation of modified BACTEC 12B radiometric medium and solid media for culture of Mycobacterium avium subsp. paratuberculosis from sheep. J Clin Microbiol 37:1077-83

Williams AF, Beck NF, Williams SP (1998) The production of EAE-free lambs from infected dams using multiple ovulation and embryo transfer. Vet J 155:79-84

Wolf, C. A. 2003. The economics of dairy production. The Veterinary Clinics of North America. Food Animal Practice 19: 271-293.

Wolfe DF, Nusbaume KE, Lauerman LH, Mysinger PW, Riddell MG, Putnam MR, Shumway LS, Powe TA (1987) Embryo transfer from goats seropositive for caprine arthritis-encephalitis virus Theriogeniology 28:307-316

Wolfe DF, Stringfellow DA, Riddell MG, Lauerman LH, Galik PK (1988) Adherence of Brucella ovis to preimplantation ovine ova Theriogeniology 30:387-393.

Woodall CJ, Mylne MJA, McKelvey WAC, Watt NJ (1993) Polymerase chain reaction (PCR) as a novel method for investigating the transmission of maedi-visna virus (MVV) by pre-implantation embryos Proc 3rd international sheep veterinary congress. Edinburgh June 1993 p 232.

Woods EJ, Benson JD, Agca Y, et al. Fundamental cryobiology of reproductive cells and tissues. Cryobiology. 2004;48(2):146-156.

Wrench N, Pinto CR, Klinefelter GR, et al. Effect of season on fresh and cryopreserved stallion semen. Animal Reproduction Science. 2010;119(3-4):219-227.

Yildiz C, Bozkurt Y, Yavas I. An evaluation of soybean lecithin as an alternative to avian egg yolk in the cryopreservation of fish sperm. Cryobiology. 2013;67(1):91-94.

York DF, Vigne R, Verwoerd DW, Querat G (1992) Nucleotide sequence of the jaagsiekte retrovirus, an exogenous and endogenous type D and B retrovirus of sheep and goats J Virol 66:4930-9

Young S (1993) Progress towards eradication of ovine progressive pneumonia from the Iowa State University teaching flocks, Proc 11th annual meeting of Iowa veterinary medical association Jan 22-24 1993

Youngs, C. R. 2011. Cryopreservation of pre-implantation embryos of cattle, sheep, and goats. J Vis Exp 54, DOI: 10.3791/2764.

Zanoni RG (1998) Phylogenetic analysis of small ruminant lentiviruses J Gen Virol 79: 1951-1961

Zhang W, Yi K, Chen C, et al. Application of antioxidants and centrifugation for cryopreservation of boar spermatozoa. Anim Reprod Sci. 2012;132(3-4):123-128.

INDEX

www.ingramcontent.com/pod-product-compliance
Lightning Source LLC
Chambersburg PA
CBHW061955190326
41458CB00009B/2879